W9-BCP-043

YOUNG CHILDREN'S BEHAVIOUR

Second Edition

YOUNG CHILDREN'S BEHAVIOUR

Practical approaches for caregivers and teachers

Second edition

Louise Porter
PhD, MA(Hons), MGiftedEd, DipEd

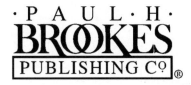

·PAUL·H·
BROOKES
PUBLISHING C? ®

Paul H. Brookes Publishing Co.
PO Box 10624
Baltimore, Maryland 21285–0624

Library of Congress Cataloging-in-Publication Data
Porter, Louise, 1958-
    Young children's behaviour: practical approaches for caregivers and teachers /
    Louise Porter.–2nd ed.
        p. cm.
    Includes bibliographical references and index.
    ISBN 1-55766-666-0
    1. Preschool children-Psychology. 2. Behavior modification. 3. Discipline of children.
    4. Early childhood education. 5. Classroom management. I. Title.
HQ774.5P67 2003
372.1102'4–dc21   2002043743

Typeset by Egan-Reid Ltd, Auckland
Printed and bound in Australia

Dedication

For my parents, Pauline Porter and Jim Porter
and grandparents, Kalvina Porter and Norman Verity
who taught me that the purpose of life
is a life with purpose.

Contents

Part One

●●

Foundations of a guidance approach

If you want to get ahead, get a theory.

With up to 800 decisions to be made by early childhood practitioners per day (Jorde-Bloom 1988), it can only help to have a rationale for these rather than having hastily to make judgments on the run—going with whatever 'seems like a good idea' at the time. Instead of this moment-by-moment decision-making, knowledge of some theory about the discipline of children would provide a coherent set of beliefs that would allow you to understand what you are aiming for, what is going on at the time of a disruption, what effects your practices are producing, and what needs changing in the event that the practices are not successful.

In advocating a system of discipline that does not use rewards and punishments, this book might appear to be asking you to adopt a new theory about children's behaviour, which might seem too onerous to be worth the effort. However, a guidance approach involves learning very little that is new. Instead, it is grounded in what you already know about teaching children all other developmental skills. When assisting toddlers to learn to walk, we do not punish them for falling over or for walking hesitantly: we encourage them, celebrate their achievements, accept mistakes as natural, and help the children to persist in the face of setbacks.

So it is with learning to behave thoughtfully. It is inevitable that children will make mistakes and act disruptively. This awareness, however, does not mean that we should tolerate inconsiderate acts and

1

passively wait for children to 'grow out of it'. Instead, we should teach them a more skilful behaviour, in the same way that we give them opportunities to improve their balance when learning to walk.

Because you already know how to teach, you already know much of what this text will tell you. But the attitudes that commonly prevail about the discipline of children often mean that we do not transfer our knowledge of teaching across to the teaching of thoughtful behaviour. The aim, then, of this book is to help you to blend the knowledge that you have about teaching developmental skills with the approaches that you use for discipline. To assist you with this, it will provide a rationale (a theory) to explain your behavioural interventions, and argue why some measures (such as punishment) should not be used. It will explain that the most powerful disciplinary tool that you have at your disposal is your caring relationship with the children. When you are sensitive to children and respond to their needs, they will develop both the skill and the desire to be sensitive to your needs in reply. This is the basis for socialising children—that is, for helping them to grow to accept their responsibilities and exercise their rights in their community.

The purpose of Part One, then, is to ground disciplinary measures within educational practice, so that how we respond to disruptions does not undo the educational aims of our wider program. Chapter 1 thus sets the scene in its discussion of the values of early years education. Next, we need to examine what we are aiming for when we discipline children, because it is much easier to reach a destination if we know where we are headed. To that end, Chapter 2 presents some debates about the discipline of children and draws some conclusions that will form the basis of the recommendations in the remainder of the book. Third, we need to appreciate that the prevention of disruptions is by far the most powerful aspect of discipline. This means that in Chapter 3 the quality of the early childhood program comes under scrutiny as the context in which we are expecting children to act thoughtfully.

Together, the chapters in Part One will present the argument that your responses to children's disruptive behaviour must:

- be consistent with the principles of high-quality early childhood care or education;
- follow the guidelines for caring interactions between adults and children in care or educational settings;
- represent ethical or just practice;

- be effective;
- promote children's skill development;
- foster children's disposition or willingness to cooperate with others;
- safeguard children's emotional needs; and
- be congruent, therefore, with the centre's broader educational goals.

Theory is often seen to be irrelevant to practice, as if practice is an art form that cannot be taught. But practitioners are disempowered by the 'craft' model in which they are handed down techniques without being trusted to comprehend the ideas that underpin these. This book aims to provide both a series of practical strategies as well as a clear rationale for their use. Only when you have both can you reflect on what is happening when a child acts disruptively and understand what to do and when.

The information given represents a compilation of the experience I have gained as a psychologist working in and consulting to preschools and child care centres; from my research study involving 200 hours of observations of disciplinary practices in child care centres, combined with interviews with caregivers; from my teaching of behaviour theory to education students at university; and from my experience as a parent. The result is a coherent set of practices with a clear theory base as a rationale.

1

- -

Core values of early childhood education

We cannot expect that [children] will profit from the incongruous messages we send when we manage for obedience and teach for exploration and risk-taking.

McCaslin and Good (1992: 13)

While structural features of child care—such as the amount of space per child, the required adult-child ratio, and maximum group size—are often laid down in local regulations or guidelines, there are very few such regulations that specify how adults should respond when children's behaviour disrupts others. Nevertheless, to receive direction, we can look to the principles that underpin our educational practices and transfer those that are pertinent into disciplinary practices.

Ethical principles

A fundamental tenet of early childhood education is that professionals must treat children and their families in an ethical fashion—that is, they must do what is right, just and good, rather than what is merely expedient, convenient or practical (Katz 1995). This generic value gives rise to some specific ethical guidelines. The first of these is *promoting the good of others*. This principle implies that, when trying to correct disruptive behaviour, any measures used must be effective. That is, they must improve the behaviour so that surrounding children or adults are protected from ongoing disruptions. Second, methods must effectively teach self-control to the children who are acting inconsiderately, so that they:

- can learn to cope with emotional setbacks without becoming overwhelmed;
- can develop pride in their ability to manage themselves; and
- do not become ostracised by others because of their inconsiderate actions.

The second principle is that you must *do no harm*. Given children's lack of power to advocate on their own behalf, you must use your influence over children in their best interests (Australian Early Childhood Association 1991). This means that you will not 'participate in practices that are disrespectful, degrading . . . intimidating, psychologically damaging, or physically harmful to children' (NAEYC 1989: 26). You must avoid punitive, humiliating or frightening disciplinary strategies and should not place unnecessary restrictions on children—that is, should not apply controls for other than safety reasons (Doherty-Derkowski 1995; NAEYC 1983).

These dual principles mean that the methods you select to correct children's disruptive behaviour must achieve the following outcomes:

- the child returns to considerate behaviour: the disruption ceases;
- the child is less likely in future to repeat the same or similar behaviour;
- the miscreant learns something positive through the process of correction, such as how to solve problems in prosocial ways;
- there are no unintended side-effects that could disadvantage the miscreant, such as increased fear of adults, feelings of intimidation, or scapegoating by peers;
- there are no spillover effects for onlookers, such as intimidation about how they would be treated if they too made a mistake;
- there are no spillover effects for adults, such as a loss of their humanity or violation of their own principles; and
- there are no deleterious effects on the adult-child relationship as a result of how a misdemeanour is handled.

The third principle is that *everyone deserves justice*—which means giving all children and families equal and fair treatment. Although this principle is usually applied with reference to characteristics such as culture, gender, religion and so on, it also requires balancing the rights and interests of one individual with those of the group. For example, although a child might have behavioural difficulties for understandable reasons such as a disability or adverse family circumstances, nevertheless you cannot expect surrounding children and adults to tolerate thoughtless behaviour. You must act to improve the child's behaviour and, if all conscientious efforts produce insufficient improvement, you must balance that child's requirements with those of others, perhaps advising parents that you cannot meet this child's needs in this setting. Allowing children to behave antisocially is not in their interests nor in the interests of others and it is unjust if one child's rights are allowed to eclipse those of surrounding individuals.

A fourth ethical principle requires that any behavioural intervention *be delivered competently* by staff with adequate training, experience and supervision.

Educational tenets

Various trends in early childhood education can be as relevant to guiding children's behaviour as they are to providing a high-quality education. These include:

- adoption of an ecological perspective that sees children's development as occurring in interaction with their environment;
- recognising development as holistic;
- a respect for pluralism and honouring of diversity;
- being responsive to children and their interests;
- focusing on the importance of learning processes—including relationships—rather than on outcomes or products;
- aiming to foster children's dispositions or willingness to learn, rather than teaching specific knowledge;
- safeguarding children's emotional wellbeing; and
- supporting parents.

An ecological perspective

Having moved away from a developmental perspective that sees children's development unfolding in some biologically-determined sequence, early childhood education increasingly has adopted an ecological perspective which states that children develop because of, rather than in, their environments (Clyde 1995). It recognises that children construct their own unique perspectives of the world, shaped by both their makeup and their social settings.

This implies that the environments we provide for children must suit their present developmental needs and context. With respect to guiding children's behaviour, it recognises that behaviour is not determined by outside rewards and punishments, but is driven by a whole constellation of internal and external factors, such as the children's home setting, their emotional needs, their problem-solving skills, the extent to which they feel accepted by peers and adults in their present setting and so on. As will be argued in Chapter 2, awareness of the complexity of human behaviour allows us to abandon a simple reward-and-punishment system of discipline in favour of one that is no more demanding on staff but takes more account of the complex factors contributing to children's behaviour.

Holism

Holism tells us that all domains of development (cognitive, language, physical, social and emotional) are interrelated (Bowman & Stott 1994). This implies that we cannot intervene in children's behaviour without regard to the impact of our corrective methods on children's other developmental skills, particularly social and emotional factors.

Pluralism

A 'melting pot' perspective includes children with an array of needs in early education, but requires the children to conform to the setting; in contrast, pluralism accepts and honours differences and adjusts the setting to fit the children's (and adults') needs (Lieber et al. 1998). This pluralistic perspective is usually discussed with reference to cultural, family and developmental differences. However, it also applies to behavioural differences. Lieber and colleagues (1998) observed that educators who seek conformity accept only a narrow range of behaviours in their young charges. This provokes the recognition that what constitutes 'misbehaviour' or 'inappropriate behaviour' is mostly defined by adults and is in the eye of the beholder (Kohn 1996). Whereas adults might interpret particular actions as unacceptable, from children's perspective, these might be understandable, given their level of reasoning skills. This does not suggest an 'anything goes' attitude to children's behaviour but raises awareness that many of the disruptive acts of children are a product of their developmental immaturity, rather than a sign of some inherent 'naughtiness'. When accepting that much of their behaviour is 'par for the course', you can correct it from a teaching rather than a moralistic or punitive stance.

Responsiveness to children's needs

There are two broad approaches to curriculum programming. The first is a *top down* approach in which adults determine which skills and information are of value to children and then set about teaching these. This approach is largely adult-driven, with educators framing programs according to their own philosophy, experience and training, beliefs about children, and aims for education. The resulting program takes account of governing policies, constraints imposed by the context or setting, and parental values and preferences. It is not necessarily unresponsive to children's needs, but is nevertheless largely originated by the educator. When this model is applied to behavioural issues, it implies that adults will determine the types of behaviours they expect of children and then shape children's behaviour to fit this mould.

In contrast, a *bottom-up* approach sees children as already enriched and vibrant human beings (Dahlberg et al. 1999) whose need to generate identities and understandings of the world are the starting point for, rather than an afterthought in, curriculum planning. In terms of guiding children's behaviour, this translates into an acceptance of where the children are presently functioning and of their need to explore social rules and mores in the same way that they explore their physical world. This, however, does not mean that you should indulge children's emotional states when their behaviour is negatively affecting others; just aim to teach them more skilful behaviour.

Focus on process rather than content

At all levels of education, processes of teaching and learning are increasingly being given more significance than *what* the children are being asked to learn. This is partly in recognition of the rapidly expanding pool of information in society, which means that knowing facts (content) is less important than knowing how to acquire them (process). When it comes to learning self-discipline, the following skills can be highlighted:

- using language to negotiate with others and to direct one's own actions;
- understanding the relationships among objects, people and events and the effects of one's actions on others; and
- practising problem-solving skills.

When educating young children, the quality of children's relationships with adults is considered the foundation for learning these skills. The same is true when disciplining children. High-quality relationships comprise adults' sensitivity to, or awareness of, children's needs, and their willingness to respond to those needs, as appropriate. These two aspects are the key to meeting some of children's need for intimacy and, in terms of guiding their behaviour, to disposing them positively to cooperate with you.

Dispositions

A key aim of early childhood education is to encourage in children positive attitudes to learning and to themselves as learners so that they remain willing to put in the effort required to achieve. These dispositions include, for example, engagement, playfulness, motivation, persistence, independence, cooperativeness, curiosity, enthusiasm for learning, confidence, patience, exploration, playfulness, adventurousness, intellectual rigour, creativity, open-mindedness, self-awareness and self-control (Lambert & Clyde 2000; Perkins et al. 1993).

With respect to children's behaviour, we must not only to make it *easier* for children to meet our expectations, but we must also make children more *willing* to do so. We need to encourage children to be considerate of others, cooperate with others, exercise self-discipline and act morally (see Chapter 2). Only when they experience us cooperating with them will they be willing to cooperate with us in return. Only when they care about us will they be disposed to considering our needs. We must relate to them in ways that do not provoke a disdain for us and instead make it more rather than less likely that in future they will treasure our good opinion of them and will seek to consider our needs as well as their own.

Emotional support for children

Early years education also aims to safeguard children's emotional development by:

- establishing a safe and caring physical and emotional environment that supports and protects all children's right to learn and grow personally;
- helping children establish satisfying and successful social relationships; and
- developing in each child a healthy self-esteem.

These emotional needs must not be violated by our disciplinary methods. For example, children must learn something positive from how they are instructed about their actions; they must be more rather than less disposed afterwards to act thoughtfully; and their self-esteem must remain intact throughout correction of their behaviour.

Support for parents

A final aim of early childhood education is to support parents (or other primary caregivers) in achieving their aspirations for their child. Unfortunately, the children with the most disruptive behaviour are often the ones with the most isolated families who are in receipt of the least external support. Ways of collaborating with parents and supporting both children and families in times of stress are outlined in Chapters 16 and 14 respectively, so will not be expanded here.

Conclusion

The methods we use to teach children and to respond to disruptive behaviour must be congruent with each other. You cannot correct a behaviour in a way that undermines what you are attempting to teach children in your wider program, or which violates their social or emotional requirements. Chapter 2 extends this argument by comparing a rewards-and-punishment system to a guidance approach to discipline, arguing that only the latter fulfils your ethical obligations to children.

Suggested further reading

Australian Early Childhood Association (1991). Australian Early Childhood Association code of ethics. *Australian Journal of Early Childhood*, 16 (1), 3-6.

National Association for the Education of Young Children (1989). Code of ethical conduct. *Young Children*, 45 (1), 25-29.

Stonehouse, A. (1991). *Our code of ethics at work*. Watson, ACT: Australian Early Childhood Association.

2

●●●

Debates about discipline

> *There is a time to admire the grace and persuasive power of an*
> *influential idea, and there is a time to fear its hold over us. The*
> *time to worry is when the idea is so widely shared that we no*
> *longer even notice it, when it is so deeply rooted that it feels to us*
> *like plain common sense. At the point when objections are not*
> *answered anymore because they are no longer even raised, we*
> *are not in control: we do not have the idea; it has us.*
>
> Kohn (1999: 3)

This chapter will contrast two styles of discipline. I shall call one a
'controlling' style because it uses rewards and punishments imposed by adults
on children—that is, it imposes control from the outside. It is the system of
discipline to which Kohn is referring in the opening quote, commenting that
the notion of rewarding 'good' behaviour and punishing undesirable actions
in order to discipline children is so widely endorsed that most of us regard it
as common sense. Many do not even realise that there are compelling
arguments against this approach and so fail to question it or look for a
better way.

The second contrasting system of discipline is called a 'guidance'
approach (Gartrell 1998). It aims to teach or guide children so that they
learn to direct their own actions—that is, from the inside. (Obviously, there
are many other theories of behaviour management but most are designed for
schools and are not applicable with very young children but, for a full review,
see Porter [2000a, 2000b].)

Contrasting philosophies

The two styles to be reviewed here have differing views on a number of issues that are central to devising disciplinary plans for young children's disruptive behaviours. These differences are summarised in Table 2.1 and include: where the theories locate individuals' control; their goals of discipline; what they regard to be the causes of behavioural disruptions; their view of children; and how they perceive behavioural mistakes (in contrast with developmental or academic mistakes). I shall now examine each of these issues in turn and conclude with what the debates imply for practice.

Locus of control

A controlling style of discipline believes that we can make others repeat behaviour of which we approve by administering a reward—that is, delivering something they value such as praise, the opportunity to do a favourite activity, stickers or 'special treats'. Correspondingly, we can decrease the likelihood that others will repeat a behaviour of which we disapprove by punishing them—that is, administering something that they don't like such as a verbal reprimand or a spanking (which, of course, is not endorsed in professional circles), or by withdrawing something that they like, such as play time or adult attention. Advice to 'reward the good and punish the bad' is based on the view that individuals' behaviour is controlled from outside themselves. In support of this contention, the controlling approach reminds us that adults work for a salary—that is, a reward—and would cease to work if they did not get paid. It is plain common sense that this is the way of the world.

In contrast, a guidance approach believes that individuals make decisions about their behaviour based on their own, internal, needs. It argues that, although aware of the regime of rewards and punishment that is in place, individuals will use this knowledge as information only. Ultimately, they will make up their own minds about whether to abide by or defy that system, depending on whether the behaviours they are contemplating meet their emotional needs (Glasser 1998). The guidance approach recognises that adults would stop working if their salary were discontinued but only because their survival (an internal need) demands that they earn an income: if they became millionaires overnight, many would still choose to do their work as they 'enjoy it'.

Other examples that are closer to home arise when you think about your own life. As an early childhood caregiver or educator, you belong to a low-paid profession. You probably knew that at the time you entered the profession but, presumably, judged that there would be rewards for you in the work itself. You might, for instance, have assessed that you could contribute something of meaning to young children's lives which, in turn, would meet your (internal) need to feel of value to others. Or, consider volunteers who give their time for no monetary reward at all. Or, consider the four-year-old who, when you enquire why he did something and ask didn't he realise that it would get him into trouble, replies 'Oh yes, I knew that. But, gee, it was worth it!'. This child is telling you that he is prepared to risk punishment to engage in a behaviour that he enjoys.

According to guidance theorists, these examples tell us that we are all controlled from within. If that is so, externally-applied rewards and punishments are virtually irrelevant, as all they provide is information: they do not determine our behaviour. Furthermore, even if individuals *can* be manipulated externally, this does not mean that they *should*. Advocates of a guidance approach contend that it is risky to use external controls, citing many disadvantages of rewards and punishments, respectively listed in Boxes 2.2 and 2.3.

The argument is sealed, in my view, by my own observations that the very children who most appear to 'need' a structured behaviour management program are the very children who are showing by their dogged refusal to cooperate with the program that it is not working and never will. They have received more (externally-applied) punishments than children with less disruptive behaviour, and still the behaviour persists. These are the children who would rather risk condemnation than sacrifice their free spirit. For the remainder—those who conform—behavioural consequences are unnecessary, as these children would cooperate anyway.

Goals of discipline

A second difference between the controlling and guidance approaches is their aims. The controlling approaches aim to teach children to comply with adult directives and, indeed, use terms such as 'non-compliance' or 'naughty' to describe behavioural difficulties. Most claim that the intent of a controlling approach is to teach children self-discipline. However, 'self-discipline' in this context often means getting children to comply with adult standards for their behaviour, regardless of whether they are being supervised or not. But this might come about only because the children are not sure when the adult will return and detect any misdeeds. This is simply internalised compliance (Kohn 1996). Instead, a guidance approach aims to teach thoughtful behaviour, which comprises:

- developing in children a sense of right and wrong so that they act considerately not because they might be punished for doing otherwise, but because it is the right thing to do. This aim could be called teaching *autonomous ethics* (Kohn 1996), in contrast with internalised compliance;
- teaching children to *regulate their emotions* so that their outbursts do not disturb those around them but, more importantly, so that they themselves learn to cope with setbacks in life;
- teaching children to *cooperate* so that all can have their needs met; and
- giving children a sense of *potency*—that is, a sense that they can make a difference to themselves and their world, can control their own actions and feelings, and can act on their values (Porter 2001).

In the vein of Calvin Coolidge's declaration that 'there is no right way to do the wrong thing' (Sapon-Shevin 1996: 196), the humanists reject the authoritarian goal of teaching obedience on the grounds that it is dangerous in three respects. First, it endangers individual children because they might not resist abuse—and here I'm thinking mainly of sexual abuse—because they have been taught to do what adults say (Briggs & McVeity 2000). Second, it is dangerous for surrounding children as those who have been trained to follow others might collude with schoolyard bullying when directed to do so by a powerful peer. Finally, whole societies would be safer if people did not follow the commands of a sociopathic leader who told them to harm members of a surrounding community whose race or religion differed from their own.

Thus, even if rewards and punishments could teach children to do as they are told, this would not be a laudable outcome. Second, rewards and punishments concentrate children's minds on what will happen *to them* if they exhibit a particular behaviour, whereas the goal of teaching children considerateness requires instead that they learn to think *of others*. So, a controlling style of discipline would actually undermine this goal.

Furthermore the goal of teaching compliance runs counter to our educational goals of empowering children to explore and grow through discovery and of teaching problem-solving skills and critical thinking (McCaslin & Good 1992). The notion of compliance is also at odds with pedagogical understandings. It assumes that infants start out as *empty vessels* or 'adults-in-waiting' who lack adult knowledge, skills, values and culture, and thus require us to correct these deficiencies (Dahlberg et al. 1999; David 1999). Achievement of this necessarily relies on adult-directed teaching and the use of behaviourist methods in which educators determine what children should know and how they should act, and then model desired skills and reinforce (reward) children for producing these.

A contrasting postmodern or *ecological* view regards children as integral parts of their various social environments, actively constructing their own experiences (Dahlberg et al. 1999). They are thus rich, inventive and competent individuals who can construct their own identities and understandings (Dahlberg et al. 1999; Fraser & Gestwicki 2002). This shifts the educational emphasis away from *telling* children what they should know and how they should behave, towards *listening* and responding to the richness of their present lives. It is clear that an ecological perspective on education cannot function cohesively alongside an 'empty vessels' notion about behaviour management.

Causes of disruptions

A controlling view of discipline believes that children's disruptive behaviour persists because, quite inadvertently, desired behaviours have been receiving too few rewards and/or undesirable behaviours have been accidentally rewarded or given insufficient punishment.

In contrast, a guidance approach locates the source of disruptions within children. It takes the view that behavioural disruptions are inevitable as children must be exuberant and explore their environment, will make mistakes because they do not yet know better or temporarily have lost control of themselves, or have learned inappropriate behaviour from others. (These reasons are outlined more fully in Chapter 7.)

More relevant to planning interventions, however, is a distinction between primary and secondary behaviours (Rogers 1998). Primary behaviours are those that arise from the drive to satisfy internal needs, as just described. Secondary behaviours are children's reactions to being disciplined. For example, in my own research into behaviour management in child (day) care centres, I noted that children who were being chastised would run away from caregivers, lash out at them, spit, swear, or destroy nearby objects while angry (Porter 1999b). Advocates of a guidance approach believe that these extreme behaviours are actually provoked by the denial of children's autonomy—that is, are a result of adults' attempts at exerting control over children externally.

This is supported by other studies that have shown that when mothers exercise restrictive control over their children, the children become defiant, uncooperative, withdrawn, anxious, unhappy, hostile when frustrated, and unwilling to persist at tasks (Baumrind 1967, 1971; Crockenberg & Litman

1990). This can be compared to authoritative parents (loosely defined as those using a guidance approach) who tend to produce children who are more cooperative, self-controlled, self-confident, independent and social. This is probably because children are more likely to cooperate with adults who have previously cooperated with them (Atwater & Morris 1988; Parpal & Maccoby 1985; Porter 1999b).

View of children

In my observations and discussions with caregivers about their practices, it became clear to me that their choice of disciplinary method related in part to their beliefs about children. We seldom make these beliefs explicit but they underpin practices all the same.

One implicit view of children is of Rousseau's *innocent child* who is seen to be basically good and will achieve virtue if uncorrupted by adult influences and permitted free and playful self-expression (Dahlberg et al. 1999). This view implies a lack of adult intervention with children for fear of 'interfering' with the natural unfolding of their process of self-discovery. With respect to discipline, this view aligns with a 'laissez-faire' or 'anything goes' approach and has no modern adherents.

The opposite, but perhaps even stronger tradition from many world religions is the notion that children are born inherently evil and that this tendency must be socialised out of them. The philosopher Thomas Hobbes once described life as nasty, brutish and short and, when it comes to responding to disruptive behaviour, it seems that some adults apply the same description to children (Kohn 1996). We give children negative labels such as naughty or noncompliant and ascribe negative motives to them such as that they are manipulative, attention-seeking or 'doing it deliberately' (perhaps even 'to get at me') but we do not use the same language to describe the behaviour of adults.

Thus, controlling methods of discipline are built on an idea that hardly anyone actually believes—which is, that children are basically 'naughty' and will try to get away with inconsiderate behaviour. If we believe this, it is a small leap to assume that they need to be directed—virtually forced—to behave well. Even though few of us believe this idea, we *act as if we do*. We praise or reward children when they behave well, as if we think that they will not act considerately again unless we 'reinforce' their behaviour. Or, we punish them when they behave in ways we do not like, as if we think they will only do it again unless we come down hard on them now.

In contrast to this 'sour' view of children (Kohn 1996) a guidance approach believes that children will behave well when treated well and poorly when disrespected. This view claims that when adults do not threaten children with punishment or bribe them with incentives for behaviour of which we approve, young people are motivated, will make constructive choices, and are more likely than not to behave thoughtfully (Kohn 1996; Rogers 1951; Rogers & Freiberg 1994).

It has been my observation that educators of young children can simultaneously hold one view—usually a positive one—when it comes to children's education and the opposite view—of inherent wickedness—when children act disruptively (Porter 1999b). This inevitably leads to differing approaches to developmental versus behavioural errors, with each undermining the other and sending mixed signals to children that they should think creatively but act obediently (McCaslin & Good 1992).

Box 2.1: Assumptions about developmental versus behavioural mistakes

Common assumptions about developmental errors	Common assumptions about behavioural mistakes
Children are trying to make the correct response.	Children are trying to be disruptive—that is, to make an *in*correct response.
Errors are accidental and inevitable.	Errors are deliberate.
Learning requires exploration.	Children should not explore limits; they should obey them.
Children who have learning difficulties need additional or modified teaching.	Children who have behavioural difficulties should be punished.

SOURCE: ADAPTED FROM JONES AND JONES (2001: 296)

Assumptions about disruptiveness

Assumptions about behavioural versus developmental mistakes are often at odds with each other, with educators commonly displaying tolerance towards children's developmental errors but a moralistic attitude towards behavioural ones, comprising notions that children 'should' or 'should not' act in particular ways (see Box 2.1). When you regard behavioural errors in this way, a controlling approach to discipline appears almost inevitable, thus incurring all of the disadvantages of rewards and punishments (see Boxes 2.2 and 2.3). In contrast, a guidance approach accepts that behavioural mistakes are as inevitable as developmental errors and so, rather than punishing children for these, will teach them how to acquire more skills. Given the inevitability of errors during childhood, if we were to punish children for making mistakes, we would be punishing them for *being* children.

Table 2.1: Summary of the difference between the controlling and guiding approaches

Discipline style	Control	Guidance
Locus of control	External	Internal
Goals	Obedience Compliance	Considerateness • autonomous ethics • regulation of emotions • cooperation with others • potency
Causes of disruptive behaviour	Insufficient rewards for desired behaviour Accidental reinforcement and/or failure to punish undesired behaviours	Normal exuberance Normal exploration Lack of skill Impaired self-control Secondary reactions to being controlled
View of children	Naturally inclined to misbehave Naughty	Will behave well if treated well and poorly if treated poorly
View of disruptive behaviour	Inappropriate Noncompliance	Natural errors An occasion for teaching
Adult's status	Boss	Leader
Intervention methods	Rewards (e.g. praise) Punishment	Acknowledgment Problem solving

Effectiveness

In Chapter 1, I introduced the notion that we must judge the effectiveness of disciplinary practices not only in light of their impact on the target behaviour but also considering their effects on the recipient, onlooking children, the adults who must correct the behaviour, and the relationship between the children and adults. Although the theories that use rewards and punishments can cite a considerable body of research demonstrating a subsequent reduction in undesired behaviours or an increase in desired ones (see Alberto & Troutman 1999; Kaplan & Carter 1995), such studies typically require highly sophisticated adjustments to reinforcers and punishers and intensive, one-to-one training of targeted children by specialists in behaviour modification. None of these conditions pertains in group-based care settings. Even then, most studies find that the behavioural improvements do not generalise—which is code for saying that, once the program ceases, the gains do too. In other words, the children have not learned from the training (Porter 1999b).

Still more relevant to the debates examined here is that these studies do not investigate whether there were side-effects on individual and surrounding children. When examining such spillover effects, my research (Porter 1999b) found that a guidance approach was both more effective at ending disruptions and avoided the negative side-effects of the rewards and punishments used by the authoritarian approaches (as summarised in Boxes 2.2 and 2.3). The conclusion, then, is that educators should guide—rather than control—children.

Box 2.2: Disadvantages of rewards

When adults determine which behaviours they approve and when and how they will deliver rewards, they clearly are in control of others. Given that exercising autonomy is a fundamental human need, violation of it carries some risks—to recipients, onlookers and administrators of rewards.

Detrimental effects on children's self-esteem
- Children will not feel accepted because they know that they are being judged.
- When ideal behaviours are rewarded, children can learn to expect themselves to 'be good' all the time, lowering their self-esteem when this is impossible.

(Continued)

Box 2.2: *(Continued)*

- Rewards teach children that other people's opinions of them are more important than their own. This can stifle self-reliance.

Rewards can impede learning
- Rewards can cause children to develop external rather intrinsic motivation.
- Children who strive for rewards might engage in 'adult watching' to assess whether adults approve of them. This will distract them from focusing on their own learning.
- Rewards cause children's performance to deteriorate: they may do more work but it is of a lower quality.
- Rewarded children might strive to please and fear making mistakes, and so avoid being creative and adventurous.

Rewards can provoke disruptive behaviour
- Discouragement about being unable to meet unrealistic expectations can cause some children to behave disruptively.
- Rewards do not teach children to monitor their own successful behaviour and so do not give them the skills to regulate their unsuccessful actions either.

Rewards can be unfair
- Adults need a high level of technical expertise to use rewards well. When praise and other rewards are misdirected, adults and their feedback lose credibility as the children realise that the reward was not justified.
- While some children 'pull' praise from adults, others do not and so receive less praise than they deserve.
- Rewards increase competition between children as they try to earn the limited number of rewards that are available and, in the process, deprive others of these.
- Their experience that praise is unfair causes some children to reject the adults who administer it.
- Many children come to resent being manipulated by rewards and behave disruptively to re-assert their autonomy.

Implications for practice

The remainder of this chapter introduces alternative practices to the use of rewards and punishments that will be enlarged on in the remainder of the book. The use of alternatives is based on the recognised disadvantages of rewards and punishments (see Boxes 2.2 and 2.3) and on the above discussion that allows us to conclude that reward and punishment strategies:

- are largely *irrelevant* as the children who most appear to need their behaviour to be adjusted are already showing that they will defy a system of rewards and punishments; while those children who are behaving cooperatively do not need manipulation in order to do so: lesser means will be successful with them;
- are *ineffective*, as rewards and punishments focus children's minds on what *they* will get out of behaving in a particular way, whereas a guidance approach seeks to teach them to focus on the effects of their behaviours *on others*;
- are *counter-productive* as controlling methods incite more difficulties than they solve and the secondary behavioural difficulties they provoke are typically severe and thus very difficult to deal with;
- are *risky* as children and controlling adults often feel dehumanised by the imposition of controls; and
- are based on a *negative view of children* which is seldom the actual view of early childhood practitioners and which contradicts their pedagogical view of children as vibrant human beings.

Box 2.3: Disadvantages of punishments

To punish children for making natural childhood mistakes would be to punish them for *being* children. Not only is this unfair, but the administration of punishment has many other drawbacks.

Limited effectiveness
- Punishment cannot prevent disruptions: children must infringe someone's rights before action is taken.
- Aversive consequences can increase undesirable behaviour.
- Children learn to behave well only to avoid punishment, rather than developing a 'conscience'.
- Adults must be constantly vigilant to detect misbehaviour, and cannot. Failure to identify the full circumstances leads to errors in administering punishment.

(Continued)

Box 2.3: *(Continued)*

- Its effects may not be permanent.
- Punishment may not replace an undesired behaviour with a more desirable one.
- Punishment works only for those who do not need it.

Detrimental effects on recipients
- Punishment can produce negative emotional side-effects, including low self-esteem.
- It can teach children to imitate exercising control over others.
- Children can learn to avoid punishing situations, either by withdrawing or by becoming submissive.
- Punishment can provoke undesirable behaviours such as resistance, rebellion, and retaliation that in turn attract more punishment.
- Punishment can intimidate onlookers even though they themselves are never punished.
- Punishment can cause onlookers to define a punished child as 'naughty' and, as a result, exclude him or her from their friendship group.

Effects on administrators and society
- Punishment can become addictive and can escalate into abuse.
- It can teach children to ignore adults who threaten but do not deliver punishment.
- Punishment damages relationships, making children less likely in future to want to please adults who use it.
- Violence in homes, care settings, preschools or schools leads to a violent and unsafe society.

Skills for guiding children

Our society has such a long tradition of trying to make children comply with our commands that the controlling approach can seem to be adults' only option. This tradition dates back so many centuries that many of us think that the term 'discipline' actually *means* 'control'. Instead, guiding skills aim to teach rather than control others. The remainder of this chapter will introduce some of the guiding skills, all of which will be explained in more detail throughout the coming chapters.

Exercise leadership

Gordon (1991) believes that adults must achieve authority by virtue of their expertise, rather than through their power to make children uncomfortable. You could think of the first style as *leadership* and the second as *bossing* (Glasser 1998). This means wisely adjusting your responses to disruptiveness in light of the circumstances at the time, in contrast with being 'consistent' in the administration of rewards or punishments.

Consider children's needs

In order to teach children to consider others, you need to begin by being sensitive to their needs and responding to those when possible. This means being tuned in to children's emotions and detecting accurately what is troubling them. This demonstrates to children how to be considerate and helps them be willing to cooperate with you some other time.

Acknowledge considerate behaviour

Most of us have been told to praise and reward children to encourage 'appropriate' behaviour. But praise is secretly manipulative: we are trying to make children do more of what we want them to do. The hidden belief is that children will not behave well naturally: they need to be forced to. But we do not reward our adult friends or tell them that they are good people when they help us out: all we do is thank them. So, we can do the same for children. They are not good people when they please us, and bad people when they displease us. It is not up to us to judge or label them, but we *can* say when we appreciate their considerate behaviour. This is a natural outcome of their actions, rather than an attempt to bribe them into repeating the behaviour again. This is discussed further in Chapter 4.

Establish guidelines, not rules

Guidelines define considerate behaviour—that is, what you want children to do (Gartrell 1998). They are reference points that make help make your responses predictable across time and different situations, but they leave you free to decide how to respond, depending on the circumstances.

In contrast, rules tell children what you *do not* want them to do and usually have predetermined penalties: 'If you do that, *this* will happen' (Gartrell 1998). Such regimented consequences leave you either having to enforce something that does not make sense in the circumstances, or appearing to be inconsistent, which will be ineffective.

Regard behavioural mistakes as natural

Most thoughtless behaviour comes about because learning to behave considerately is a developmental task, just like any other that children must acquire—albeit far more complex than other developmental skills. Just as children need to learn how to walk, so too they need to learn how to be considerate. And just as we would not punish toddlers for falling over, so too we should not punish children for behavioural mistakes. Mistakes are natural at all ages, and are an occasion for teaching children how to be more skilful, rather than a reason to punish.

Resolve problems through communication

When children are acting in ways that disrupt others, a guidance approach calls on you to look for a solution rather than a culprit (Gordon 1970). Solving the problem will involve listening, being assertive, and using collaborative problem-solving skills. These are all detailed in Chapter 7.

Teach self-control

We would regard it as strange if a first-year teacher complained that the children in his or her class could not read or write. It is strange, because that is normal for young children. But we would be dismayed if the teacher then announced a plan to wait around to see if the children figured it out for themselves: we would expect a teacher to teach skills that we know are useful for children.

So it is with behaviour. Young children cannot know how to behave considerately all the time—but that does not mean we should tolerate inconsiderateness and hope that they will learn better eventually. Just as with learning any other skill, we should set about teaching it.

Nevertheless, this might not mean teaching the skill itself but teaching children how to regain command of themselves so that they can exercise a skill that is already in their repertoire. Mostly, we assume that when children are not able to behave considerately, this is because they do not know how to do so. Instead, in my observations, most children know how they should be acting but temporarily are overwhelmed by their feelings and cannot act on that information. Methods to help them regain self-control are outlined in Chapter 9.

Conclusion

Discipline will only ever safeguard individual children from abuse, and protect society from the behavioural excesses of its members, when individuals accept responsibility for themselves and can seek to satisfy their own needs without violating the needs of other people. In the early childhood years the goal of discipline, then, is to give children the confidence to take increasing responsibility for their own actions and for the effect of these on other people.

In this chapter I have argued that we can achieve the same—actually, better—behavioural outcomes by means other than rewards and punishments, with few of the risks associated with the controlling style of discipline. The guiding skills introduced here, and enlarged upon in coming chapters, can be very similar to their controlling counterparts and so can involve virtually the same responses as you presently use, but with a difference in flavour or style. Your intent will be to guide or teach rather than to manipulate children. In turn, children will detect this difference and will respond differently to the two methods, displaying fewer secondary behavioural difficulties when their autonomy is not being denied.

Suggested further reading

To examine the range of theories of behaviour management, you could refer to:

Porter, L. (2000). *Student behaviour: Theory and practice for teachers.* (2nd ed.) Sydney: Allen and Unwin; or its equivalent title, *Behaviour in schools: Theory and practice for teachers.* Buckingham, UK: Open University Press.

For further discussion of a guidance approach to discipline:
Gartrell, D. (1998). *A guidance approach for the encouraging classroom.* New York: Delmar.
Gordon, T. (1991). *Teaching children self-discipline at home and at school.* Sydney: Random House.
Kohn, A. (1996). *Beyond discipline: From compliance to community.* Alexandria, VA: Association for Supervision and Curriculum Development.
Kohn, A. (1999). *Punished by rewards: The trouble with gold stars, incentive plans, A's, praise and other bribes.* (2nd ed.) Boston, MA: Houghton Mifflin.

3

• •

Prevention of inconsiderate behaviour

> *We need young adults who can think and act creatively, who value human life, are able to make discerning decisions, and know how to communicate and negotiate rather than fight. It is our responsibility as guardians of these values to establish learning environments that foster freedom and responsibility.*
>
> ROGERS (1994: IV)

With some infants attending child care for only 500 fewer hours than they will attend school (NCAC 1993), child care and—to a lesser extent—preschool is a 'home away from home' for the young children present. Whereas once child care was seen as a compensation for home care that was deemed inadequate, or as a necessary (but not desirable) way to allow parents of young children to return to the paid work force, nowadays, early childhood centres are increasingly seen to be places *for* children whose dual role is to provide educational experiences that complement the learning children gain elsewhere and to support the community (Dahlberg et al. 1999; Moss 1999). This modern focus means that we are obliged to design settings that meet children's needs. This is valuable as an end in itself and will also prevent those avoidable behavioural difficulties that can arise when children's needs are not being met.

Provide a child-friendly environment

The physical arrangement of the centre has many behavioural effects. First, the environment affects the participation of the children by its level of stimulation, attractiveness and fun. When children are actively engaged, they are less likely to find disruptive things to do (as well as being more likely to enjoy their participation). Second, the environment can help children to feel safe and it can give them confidence that they can exercise choice and be independent and so have control of themselves during their play. Third, the layout of the centre allows the program to flow smoothly, for example, by keeping traffic areas free of congestion. Providing sufficient space avoids the unintentional collisions that can occur when children are in close proximity to each other, as well as avoiding 'deliberate' aggression and promoting cooperation (Lady Gowrie Child Centre Melbourne 1987).

This point is made clearly by Sebastian (1987: 95):

> The environment and how it is planned is a powerful regulator of behaviours. Like language it communicates clear messages of intent and feeling . . . A carefully planned environment can foster in children and adults a sense of support and control; safety and trust; independence and choice; and stimulation and challenge.

Adult-child ratio

Although an accepted canon of early years education is that there should be high numbers of adults to children, the presence of more adults is beneficial only as long as it results in a higher quality and rate of interactions between adults and children, rather than simply increased supervision (Tizard et al. 1976) or increased chat between adults (Goodnow 1989). Furthermore, when extra adults are available to assist children with additional needs it is important that adults not shadow those children constantly and thus create dependency or act as a barrier between the children and peers (Hauser-Cram et al. 1993).

Group size

The size of a group will either enable or hinder personal interactions between group members. Groups could have one adult to five children (with a total group size of six people) or three adults to 15 children, which maintains the same adult-child ratio but yields a group size of 18 members. The dynamics in these two groups will differ considerably, with very young children and perhaps older children with developmental delays being less able to cope well in a larger group. To avoid behavioural disruptions, such children may require smaller groups, particularly at times when their skills are being extended such as during group story time, or when group size imposes extended waiting time on children with limited concentration.

Having said this, a large group seems to be most detrimental when caregivers are attempting to impose external controls on the children (Porter 1999b). This style of discipline becomes particularly ineffective when there are too many children to oversee; whereas staff using a guidance approach tend to be able to manage a larger group. This might be because guidance fosters autonomous cooperation in the children or because those caregivers who tend to use a guidance approach satisfy the children's curricular and emotional needs, thus avoiding disruptions that arise when these are not met.

As long as you can be aware of the children who cannot engage without support and mediate their involvement, and can use a guidance approach to discipline, a bigger group size (space and equipment permitting) does not have to be disadvantageous. Nevertheless, we must keep in mind that even if the room is large enough to accommodate more children, young children are not developmentally ready to accommodate a crowd.

It is also worth mentioning that groups can be too small. Perhaps there are a handful of children who do not have an afternoon nap, or your centre has few children in attendance on a particular day. My observations have been that a smaller group can find it difficult to engage with activities, as if there needs to be a minimum number of children to increase the chances that one of them will be able to instigate some play in which the others can participate (Porter 1999b).

Age mix of the children

Grouping refers to the span of ages and developmental levels within a group. Groups containing children of widely differing ages pose some particular challenges for programming. It is acknowledged to take more skill to run a vertical group than a horizontal one (Mason & Burns 1996). If the programming challenges are not satisfactorily overcome, the rate of disruptions within the group is likely to increase.

Heterogeneous (also known as mixed-age, mixed-ability or vertical) grouping affects the curriculum. For instance, equipment that is suitable for the older children can be dangerous for the younger ones and so there is a risk of 'dumbing down' the curriculum to make it safe for the younger children. The result can be that the older children are deprived of the advanced activities that they need in order to feel challenged so, with little else to occupy them, they may become disruptive. Meanwhile, younger children may be vulnerable to discouragement or disengagement as a result of activities being too difficult for them.

Thus, although vertical grouping offers some social and educational benefits for children and fosters a climate of acceptance of diversity (see

Bouchard 1991; Katz et al. 1990; Lloyd 1997; Mosteller et al. 1996; Roberts et al. 1994; Veenman 1995, 1996) its effects on the children's behaviour must also be taken into account when planning group composition.

Meet children's emotional and social needs

This is the topic of Part Two of this book so will not be discussed here, except to say that when children's behaviour disrupts others in the group, your approach will affect how safe the children—both those being disciplined and onlookers—feel in the centre, and whether they develop trust in their fair treatment by adults. Therefore, as mentioned in Chapter 1, corrective measures must do more than reinstate order but must uphold children's emotional needs as well.

Provide an individually appropriate program

Although the focus of this book is on guiding young children's behaviour, that does not occur in a vacuum. A stimulating curriculum is a means of meeting children's physical, psychological, social, intellectual and academic needs (Greenberg 1992); a secondary aim is to engage children so that they do not find alternative, less productive things to do, resulting in disruptions to others.

Having listed in Chapter 1 the aims of early childhood curricula, it is worth repeating here those that most relate to the prevention of behavioural disruptions:

- develop children's enthusiasm for learning;
- impart self-management skills to children;
- facilitate the development of higher-order thinking and problem-solving skills;
- help children to establish satisfying and successful social relationships; and
- develop in each child a healthy self-esteem.

It is self-evident that these aims apply across all domains and processes, which includes disciplinary practices. It was argued in Chapter 2 that discipline must aim to educate children in moral decision-making rather than simply make them conform to adult standards. This is not only because of the risks of teaching conformity, but because early childhood programs aim to teach children how to learn and think, and this aim cannot co-exist with the aim of teaching them to do as they are told—that is, without thinking about the issue and weighing it up for themselves.

Your program or curriculum will need to encourage active participation, provide a variety of appropriate learning activities and build on and reflect individual children's physical, psychological, social, intellectual and academic needs and readinesses (Greenberg 1992). By being responsive in this way to the children's interests and needs, your curriculum will not only be developmentally appropriate but also, 'humanly, culturally and individually appropriate' (Stonehouse 1994a: 76) and, in meeting children's needs will promote their productive engagement.

Provide sufficient equipment

The most obvious way to prevent disputes over play equipment is to make sure that you have numerous items of the same toy so that children do not have to wait too long for a turn. Another is to provide two equally attractive activities in parallel so that, if a child has his or her heart set on participating in a particular activity but there is no room, at least an equally appealing option is available in the interim.

Establish some routines

Routines that are aimed at helping the day run smoothly will ultimately promote the comfort, health and wellbeing of the children. Routines help young children know what will happen next and to understand what they have to do. With this knowledge, the children's observance of a routine will require less adult supervision. Therefore, routines both help you, and give the children a sense of control. On the other hand, you must also be willing to adjust routines in response to changed circumstances or the children's needs. Otherwise, your enforcement of a routine that does not make sense to the children will pit you against them, in turn creating resistance in the children at having to abide by your directives.

A second issue is that routines must offer choice, while still enabling the children to execute what is required of them. For example, when the activity is demanding—as is the case at meal times—caregivers need to reduce the demands that the process makes on children and on themselves. Some suggestions for achieving this are given in Chapter 11.

Minimise waiting time

It is important to plan how children will move between activities so that waiting time is minimised. If we want children to learn to be considerate, adults have to be considerate of them: making children wait is both disrespectful and an invitation to behavioural difficulties as disengaged children will move off-task to entertain themselves.

Balance active and calming activities

Children need to release pent-up energy through regular physical activity while, at other times, they might need some calming activities so that their behaviour does not become disorganised. This is particularly true of children with sensory integration difficulties but is vital for all children in general.

Cater for children with additional needs

It will be important for you to recognise when children's development is not proceeding as expected so that early intervention can minimise the impact of their developmental anomalies on other aspects of their lives. This requires that you have a process for assessing children's skills. This will be particularly detailed when children have atypical needs but otherwise might involve routine observations of all the children, referring to a developmental chart to check that their skills are progressing as expected.

In response to children's additional needs, their program might require some adjustment so that they can experience success and circumvent their limitations (see Chapter 14). Elements of the program that could need modification are (Porter 2002a, 2002b):

- aspects of the *environment*—such as the arrangement of play areas, adult-child ratios or group composition;
- teaching *processes*—including increased adult instruction or mediation of children's play and learning; and
- program *content*—with adjustments aimed at ensuring that tasks are attainable by the children.

Safeguard children's health

Children can become anxious and will act up if they *feel* unwell. Chronic ear infections, medication side-effects, poor diet, lack of sleep, being over- or under-weight, or food sensitivities can upset children physically so that they cannot cope with any additional stresses. When already physically stressed, they can seem to over-react to minor irritations, thus giving the appearance of a behavioural difficulty, when instead they need medical help. If you think this could apply to individual children in your care, you might suggest that their parents arrange for a medical assessment.

Adjust demands

Prevention works at two levels: avoiding the occurrence of disruptions in the first place; and preventing their escalation or recurrence once difficulties are surfacing. When a problem is brewing, you can change the demands of the situation so that difficulties never eventuate. For example, when children are whizzing down the path on bikes at such speed as to endanger themselves or others in the playground, you could create an obstacle course that both prevents accidents by slowing the children down and makes the game more interesting. This means that the children still get their needs met and are able to enjoy their activity, while you still meet your need to provide a safe environment.

Conclusion

The above measures recognise that there are many factors making it difficult for children to behave as we would like. Thus, you will need to take charge of those that are within your control so that you make it possible—even probable—that children will act thoughtfully. It cannot be emphasised enough that, when individual children are acting thoughtlessly, you *must* examine the context where they are presently functioning and make adjustments to the program to *enable* more considerate behaviour and you *must* develop caring relationships with troublesome children, in order to make them more *willing* to cooperate with you. No behavioural intervention—no matter how skilfully employed—can compensate for a program that does not meet children's developmental, social and emotional needs.

Suggested further reading

The following texts outline effective programming approaches aimed at meeting children's developmental needs across all domains:

Bredekamp, S. & Copple, C. (Eds.) (1997). *Developmentally appropriate practice in early childhood programs.* (rev. ed.) Washington, DC: National Association for the Education of Young Children.

Fraser, S. & Gestwicki, C. (2002). *Authentic childhood: Exploring Reggio Emilia in the classroom.* Albany, NY: Delmar.

MacNaughton, G. & Williams, G. (1998). *Techniques for teaching young children: Choices in theory and practice.* Sydney: Longman.

National Association for the Education of Young Children website: http://www.naeyc.org

Part two

∙ ∙

Children's emotional needs

> We want more for our children than healthy bodies. We want our children to have lives filled with friendship and love and high deeds. We want them to be eager to learn and be willing to confront challenges . . . We want them to grow up with confidence in the future, a love of adventure, a sense of justice, and courage enough to act on that sense of justice. We want them to be resilient in the face of the setbacks and failures that growing up always brings.

SELIGMAN (1995: 6)

Children's emotional needs have been categorised differently by various authors, but a composite list could comprise:

- security—an assurance of physical and emotional protection and safety;
- self-esteem—the need to value themselves;
- autonomy—the need to be self-determining and to have some freedom;
- belonging—the need to love and be loved;
- fun—the 'intangible joy' that probably arises from the satisfaction of the above needs (Glasser 1998: 30); and
- self-expression (or self-actualisation)—the need to utilise our abilities fully and fulfil our mission in life.

Any chosen disciplinary measures must safeguard these emotional needs—both for the children's wellbeing and also to avoid provoking behavioural outbursts that arise when children's needs are frustrated or blocked. This is affirmed by the National Childcare Accreditation Council (1993: 10) which states that discipline must 'always encourage the individuality and confidence of children and never lower their self-esteem'.

To that end, the two chapters in this section give some recommendations for meeting children's emotional needs while teaching considerate behaviour. It was argued in Part One that a guidance approach could achieve both.

4

• •

Meeting children's emotional needs

Self-esteem is not a trivial pursuit that can be built by pepping children up with empty praise, extra pats, and cheers of support. Such efforts are temporary at best, and deceptive at worst. Our children need coaches, not cheerleaders.

CURRY AND JOHNSON (1990: 153)

Meeting children's emotional needs is crucial for three reasons. First and foremost, it is important in its own right as one of the main means of helping children to be well-adjusted. Second, by responding to what children require emotionally, we are equipping them to consider us in return—we have shown them how, and we have made them positively disposed to doing so. Third, in terms of this book's emphasis on behavioural disruptions, failure by children to regulate their emotions will lead to behavioural outbursts. Together, these rationales mean that satisfying children's emotional needs will help both them and surrounding individuals as the children are more likely to act thoughtfully.

In this chapter, I shall discuss the three emotional needs for safety, autonomy and self-esteem. Social needs will be discussed in Chapter 5. The longest section in this chapter covers self-esteem but that by no means indicates that it is more important—perhaps, however, more complex—than the other emotional needs.

Safety and security

Adults can choose to take part in activities and to associate with people who bolster our self-esteem, but children are at the mercy of the contexts in which we place them (Katz 1995). This means that they rely on you to create an accepting environment in which they can feel emotionally safe and confident about their ability to meet the demands being placed on them. Some means of doing so include the following.

- Require children to act considerately so that surrounding children are not intimidated by the out-of-control behaviour of a peer, and to teach miscreants skills that they can be proud of.
- Prohibit put-downs by others (see Chapter 12).
- Encourage children to be assertive when their needs are being disregarded so that they do not feel at the mercy of others. Follow up if their assertive message is not causing the offender to desist (see Chapter 7).
- Be alert for signs of child abuse (see Chapter 14).
- Use a guidance approach to discipline so that children are not taught simply to do as they are told and therefore can learn that they can resist abuse.

Autonomy

The next emotional need is for independence or autonomy, which means being governed by oneself (Kamii 1985). It amounts to learning to trust oneself. When children have autonomy and competence, they develop a healthy self-esteem (Coopersmith 1967) and a sense of initiative. In contrast, when children are controlled by adults, they may become hostile at this violation of their basic need to be self-determining (Ginott 1972). Thus, a fundamental aim of a guidance approach to discipline is to satisfy children's need for self-determination.

Give children choices

Involve children in making decisions that affect them, as they need repeated opportunities to exercise choices, use initiative and be self-determining. Asking for their suggestions and listening to their ideas tells them that you value them and believe in their abilities to take responsibility for themselves.

On the other hand, it is important not to *ask* children to participate when there is no choice *whether* to do so. But you can still give them a choice of *how* to go about it. For example, at pack-up time, you would not ordinarily ask if children want to help pack away, but could ask if they would like to pack away the blocks or the paints.

Teach children to take responsibility for outcomes

Teach children to take responsibility for the effects of their behaviours so that they learn that *they* are in command of their decisions and actions. Three measures can encourage this.

- As children will need to *experience* success, rather than simply be *told* that they are successful, you should give feedback that is both genuine and specific. That is, you should not tell children that they have been successful when they have not, and should give feedback that is specific enough for them to be able to act on the information you have given.
- Allow children to experience both success *and* failure, so that they can form a link between their actions and the outcome (Seligman 1975). If they are always successful, no matter what they do, they will feel just as helpless as if they are always fail, no matter what they do.
- To encourage them to persist in the face of setbacks, you will need to teach children to attribute the outcome to their own effort, rather than to uncontrollable factors such as inability or luck. This is called attribution training. It involves guiding children to: define failures as *temporary* rather than permanent; as *specific* to the event rather than a sign of a general or all-pervasive failing on their part; and in terms of their *behaviour*, not personality: they need to take personal responsibility without taking blame (Seligman 1995). So, without confronting them with their mistakes, you should not allow them to make excuses or teach them to do so by blaming a 'naughty' step for tripping them over, for example, but instead might comment that they forgot to watch out for the step.

Minimise stress

Strictly speaking, stress is a physical reaction to feeling out of control, particularly of negative events in life, in contrast with worries which are the cognitive component, and anxiety which is the emotional aspect of distress. However, in common usage, the word 'stress' is usually a shorthand way of referring to all three aspects. Children whose families are stressed can become overwrought themselves (see Chapter 14), while children who have emotional or behavioural difficulties can themselves create stress in those around them, which then rebounds on them (Luthar & Zigler 1991).

You can support stressed children, first, by noticing the signs of stress such as behavioural acting out or withdrawal and allowing children to discuss their feelings. Second, you can assist children to solve challenges in ways that enhance their self-confidence, promote mastery and encourage them to take appropriate responsibility for themselves (Rutter 1985).

You must ensure that your program does not provoke stress and consequent disruptions by imposing expectations that the children feel unable to meet. Meanwhile, the structure of the program—say, the balance of active versus passive activity, or the group size—must not be too demanding.

Provide extra support for stressed children

You will need to compensate for the extra pressures of some children's lives by increasing the amount of support you give them, so that they can continue to grow as people. It is harder now for children to grow up feeling confident about the many skills they are expected to master at such young ages (Curry & Johnson 1990)—particularly when some of their worries are really adult responsibilities (see Chapter 14).

Self-esteem

The third emotional need to be discussed in this chapter is for a healthy self-esteem. Erikson (1963) and Lipsitz (1984) (both in Jones & Jones 2001) believe that children—especially young children—need to see themselves as competent, and to have this competence expanded and verified by other people who are important to them.

In their first two years or so, when young children are learning to trust their caregivers, their self-esteem relies almost entirely on whether they feel loved and *accepted*. After that age, their self-esteem begins to be fed by how much *control* they can exercise over their lives: hence their determined cries of, 'I do it by myself'. They use adults' reactions to their attempts at independence to judge if they should feel pleased—that is, *morally virtuous*—or guilty about their efforts, and they begin to define themselves as *competent* or as failures (Curry & Johnson 1990).

So, self-esteem is learned. Adults' reactions tell children about the type of people they are, which builds into a picture of themselves (known as the self-concept). Others' reactions also feed their ideals which prescribe the type of people we want them to be. The comparison between these two aspects—the self-concept and ideal self—constitutes self-esteem, which becomes a measure of how we achieve our ideals. That is, self-esteem has three parts (Burns 1982; Pope et al. 1988), as shown in Figure 4.1.

Figure 4.1: Diagram of self-esteem as the overlap between the self-concept and ideal-self

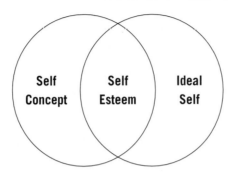

The self-concept

This is our picture or description of ourselves. This aspect is also termed self-perceptions. Young children's self-concept is fairly basic and becomes more comprehensive as they grow older and learn more about themselves. At young ages, they tend to describe themselves according to how they look, what they wear, their state of health and their possessions. As they get older, they begin to describe their relationships within and outside the family (which includes ancestors as well as living people), abilities and talents at sport and academic work, temperament, religious ideas, and ability to manage their own lives (Sekowski 1995; van Boxtel & Mönks 1992). These characteristics span five facets: social, emotional, academic, family, and physical which together form a global or overall self-concept (Pope et al. 1988; van Boxtel & Mönks 1992). Each of these aspects is also divided into sub-facets which are more situation-specific and so equate with 'self-confidence' (van Boxtel & Mönks 1992).

The ideal self

The ideal self is a set of beliefs about how we 'should' be. We learn these standards from actual or implied critical judgments by significant people in our lives or by a process called social comparison, in which we compare ourselves to other people and evaluate ourselves accordingly (Adler et al. 2001).

Self-esteem

Not all the characteristics that we possess are equally important to us. Feedback from others allows us to rank our characteristics according to how important or valued they are to other people and we usually internalise those value systems. The self-esteem, then, reflects how much we *value* our characteristics. It is a judgment about whether our abilities and qualities meet or fall short of the standards we believe are ideal. A mathematical way of saying this, then, could be (Mruk 1999):

$$Self\text{-}esteem = \frac{perceived\ success}{aspirations}$$

Being calculated in this way, it becomes clear that individuals' self-esteem can change if either their perception of their successes changes, or they adjust their aspirations or ideals (Mruk 1999).

Signs of low self-esteem

Individuals with a healthy self-esteem are realistic about their shortcomings but not harshly critical of them (Pope et al. 1988). They have a relatively balanced perception of their positive qualities and realistic expectations of themselves. As a result, they have a high degree of overlap between how they think they are and how they want to be, as depicted in Figure 4.1. (The self-concept and ideal self will never overlap entirely, of course, otherwise individuals would have no ambitions or goals for which to strive: most emotionally healthy individuals believe that they have around three-quarters of the characteristics they would like to have.)

Box 4.1 catalogues the common characteristics of children with a healthy self-esteem. In contrast with this list, children who have low self-esteem can display a wide range of less adaptive behaviours. Because they do not believe that they are valued for themselves, they might constantly try to earn adult approval through being overly helpful, repeatedly declaring affection for others (seeking a return declaration), or reacting hysterically to any real or implied criticism. They might display immature behaviours, such as un-realistic fears.

Socially, children with low self-esteem might not be able to have any fun, can be withdrawn and might be too self-conscious or 'shy' past the usual age. Finding and keeping friends can be a problem, and negotiating conflict can be difficult because they do not have enough confidence to defend themselves. They might be bullied on the one hand, or easily led on the other.

In terms of their learning, children who doubt their abilities often avoid trying something new, avoid taking risks or being adventurous, and give up easily. Instead, they might play the same game over and over—such as playing only in the sandpit—because they are afraid that they would fail at everything else. They can get very frustrated with their mistakes and so prefer to avoid new challenges than risk doing something wrongly. They will lack initiative and be uncertain about making decisions.

In its most extreme form, the low self-esteem of abused children arises from the deeply-set belief that they are unlovable (see Chapter 14). As a result, even in their preschool years they can display self-destructive, risky, or self-mutilating behaviours, including having suicidal fantasies.

Box 4.1: Characteristic behaviours of children with a healthy self-esteem

When children have a healthy self-esteem they:

- make transitions easily
- approach new and challenging tasks with confidence
- set goals independently
- have a strong sense of self-control
- assert their own point of view when opposed
- trust their own ideas
- initiate activities confidently
- show pride in their work and accomplishments
- cope with (occasional) criticism and teasing
- tolerate frustration caused by mistakes
- describe themselves positively
- make friends easily
- lead others spontaneously
- accept the opinions of other people
- cooperate and follow rules, remaining largely in control of their own behaviour
- make good eye contact (although this will vary across cultures)

SOURCES: ADLER ET AL. 2001; CLARK 1997; CURRY & JOHNSON 1990

Routes to low self-esteem

Self-esteem is both a *cause* of future learning and a *result* of achieving below expectations at relevant and worthwhile activities. This awareness points to the first cause of low self-esteem—namely, when individuals do *not have the skills* that they value.

A second route to an unhealthy self-esteem is when individuals have many valued skills and qualities but *do not realise it*. They do not appreciate their skills: their self-concept is impoverished. These children need more information about their attributes.

Third, some people have *standards that are just too high*. Gifted children, for instance, can be prone to this (see Chapter 13). In that case, you do not want to teach them to lower their standards as their perfectionism is the engine that drives them to achieve, but you do need to give them confidence that they can reach their ideals. You might also have to teach them to distinguish which things are worth doing well and which do not matter.

Facilitating children's healthy self-esteem

These three ways in which children can develop low self-esteem imply three routes for improving how they feel about themselves: helping children become competent at skills that they value, embellishing their self-concept, and ensuring that their ideals are reasonable.

Promote children's competence

Children will feel best about themselves and their abilities when they are meeting meaningful challenges and putting in some real effort (Katz 1995). Success at something meaningful breeds confidence. So, when children are not acquiring skills and qualities that are worthwhile, they do not benefit from attempts to placate them with messages like, 'There, there, it doesn't matter'. Instead we need to help them to achieve their goals so that they *can* feel proud of themselves. Therefore, the children will need specific coaching to develop competencies that they value.

Encourage children to be independent. It is important for their self-esteem that children acquire skills such as being able to separate from their parents and performing self-care tasks at an appropriate age. Sometimes, our good intentions to help children mean that we do something for them that they could do for themselves. Instead, let children attempt tasks for themselves, even if they make mistakes along the way, so that they develop faith in their ability to learn and are willing to take risks.

Teach self-instruction skills. Success at tasks involves not only being able to perform the skill, but also being able to organise oneself to do it proficiently. Therefore, teach children how to concentrate, plan each step of a task, check that their approach is working, persist, change approaches if necessary and so on.

Require considerate behaviour. Being able to control their own behaviour will also give children a skill to feel proud about.

Embellish children's self-concept

Our self-esteem—the comparison of our performance with our ideals—has both an intellectual and an emotional component (Pope et al. 1988). That is to say, how we *think* about our achievements affects how we *feel* about them. If our thinking highlights our deficiencies and ignores our achievements, our emotional reactions to our supposed deficiencies are likely to be unrealistic or 'over the top'.

Therefore, it is important for children to have a realistic picture of themselves. Many children know their limitations but take their abilities for granted and, as a result, have low self-esteem. This makes it important to give them information about themselves so that they can develop a comprehensive picture of their skills and qualities.

Acknowledgment. I believe that the single most powerful way that you can help children to develop a healthy self-esteem is to acknowledge and celebrate their successes, without praising these. Children need *information* about their attainments—as that will embellish their self-concept—but *judgmental* feedback in the form of praise tells them about what you regard as ideal behaviour. This evaluative feedback feeds their ideal self, raising their standards, perhaps to a point where they feel that they can seldom attain what you expect of them. The circles in Figure 4.1 will separate further apart.

Acknowledgment differs from praise in the following ways:

1. Acknowledgment teaches children to evaluate their own efforts: *'What do you think of that?'*. . . *'Was that fun?'*. . . *'Are you pleased with yourself?'*. . . *'You seem pleased that you did that so well'*. In comparison, praise approves of work that meets adult standards.

2. Unlike praise, acknowledgment does not judge children or their work, although you could give them your opinion of their achievement. For example, *'I like the colours you used'*, replaces the judgment that a painting is 'beautiful'.

3. Acknowledgment is a private event that does not show children up in public or compare them with each other. Unlike praise, it does not try to manipulate other children into copying a child who has been praised. Acknowledgment simply describes—in private—what the adult appreciated: *'Thanks for sitting quietly today in group time: it helped the other children to enjoy the story'*, or, *'I appreciate that you helped pack the toys away'*.

> **Guiding principle**
> If you want children to develop a healthy self-esteem, stop praising
> them.

Of course, you can still tell children that they are terrific, although not
for doing something that pleases you, but simply because they *are* wonderful.
The reason you tell them that they are terrific is to let them know that you
care for them; praise, on the other hand, tries to make them be a particular
kind of person.

Many people argue that praise is well-intentioned so perhaps it has few
disadvantages in reality, and that anyway it is too difficult to change from
praising to acknowledging children. They might argue that it did not harm
them to have been praised as children, and some even say that they continue
as adults to like receiving praise. My responses are, first, that praise does not
always have negative effects but that *it is risky*. It is particularly risky when
children are young and forming their personality: if from a young age all they
learn is that they must meet others' standards or risk disapproval, they will
have no practice at developing their own standards. Second, if you expect
to receive a reward—such as a Christmas bonus in your pay packet—and do
not, it *feels like a punishment*. This tells us that rewards and punishments are
two sides of the same coin so both can have detrimental effects, whatever
the intentions of those delivering them. Third, if tempted to use a guidance
style while continuing to use praise, you are leaving out a key ingredient of
that approach. Just as you would not expect a cake to turn out according to
the recipe if you left out the eggs or baking powder, so too a guidance
approach based on adult delivery of rewards (including praise) will not
produce children who can decide right from wrong independently of adult
supervision.

Fourth, learning to acknowledge children actually is not difficult. You
already know how to do it as you acknowledge—rather than praise—the
adults in your life. If a friend completed a training course, you would not say
'Well done! That's terrific' or even 'Good girl. That's great' but would
congratulate her and, perhaps, comment that what she has achieved
was very difficult. When a friend has helped you out by, say, picking up
your children from school when your car broke down, you would not say
'You're a good friend' but instead 'Thank you. I am really grateful that you
could help'.

So the examples in Box 4.2 illustrating the distinction between praise and acknowledgment avoid one-up-one-down language in which you are the expert and have a right to judge others and their performances. Instead, acknowledgment allows children to monitor and assess their own performances, and thus to develop a comprehensive picture of their own skills and qualities. A secondary benefit is, now that they know how to notice their behaviour, they are able to recognise when it is less successful as well, and so self-monitoring is a valuable disciplinary tool as well as a key means to foster children's healthy self-esteem.

Box 4.2: Examples of praise versus acknowledgment

Action:	A child has helped pack up the play equipment.
Praise:	You're a good helper.
Acknowledgment:	Thanks for your help.
	I appreciate your help.
	Thanks, that's made my job easier.
Plus information:	Thanks for packing away so quickly. Now there is more time to play outside.
	Thanks for packing away when I asked. That way I did not have to ask over and over, which is nicer for you and for me.
Comment:	Children usually cannot infer the effects of their actions on others and so, compared with adults, might need some additional information so that they are clear why you appreciated their behaviour.
Action:	After much effort, a child has built a tall tower of blocks.
Praise:	Well done! That's terrific!
Acknowledgment:	Congratulations!
	Wow! Look at *that*!
	Hey, you did it!
	You look very pleased with that!
Specific feedback:	I'm impressed that you kept trying even though the blocks fell over so often.

(Continued)

Box 4.2: *(Continued)*

	I admire that you figured out that the bigger blocks had to be at the bottom.
	I see that you're proud of your tower. I agree with you: I think you deserve to be.
Comment:	As we are trying to encourage in children dispositions such as persistence, problem-solving and exploration, these are the very qualities that we can comment on when we deliver informative (not judgmental) feedback so that they hear specific information about their achievements. Although they might be too young to understand words such as 'respect', 'impressed', or 'admire', as is the case with all their language learning, by interpreting the context, children soon come to know what these words convey.
Action:	The child has completed a painting and comes to you asking 'Is this good?'
Praise:	Hey, that's great! Good for you.
Acknowledgment:	You look delighted with that! I agree with you, I think you should be pleased.
	Looks like you enjoyed doing that.
	You seem disappointed with it.
Discussion:	Tell me about . . .
	What part of it don't you like?
	How come it didn't turn out as you'd hoped?
	What's your favourite part?
	It looks to me like you planned your painting very carefully.
Comment:	Children who are trying to 'pull' praise from adults are thirsty for some emotive feedback. Only after their emotions have been validated will they be interested in any specific discussion about their achievement.

(Continued)

Box 4.2: *(Continued)*

Action:	A child has reluctantly shared an item of play equipment with a playmate.
Praise:	Good boy for sharing.
Acknowledgment:	Thanks for sharing with Sam. She looked sad that she had nothing to play with.
	Sam seems really grateful that you let her have a turn.
	I appreciate that you gave Sam a turn. That way everyone can have some fun.
Comment:	In this instance, acknowledgement is focusing on the effect of the thoughtful behaviour on its recipient.

Make your feedback specific. Acknowledgment will teach children to notice their own qualities, especially if you give specific and repeated feedback about behaviours or qualities that you value in children. At the same time, keep in mind that children's self-esteem will depend on the extent to which they make the most of their potential. If you praise children for inherited characteristics, their self-esteem is not likely to improve, as they had no control over those characteristics. So you will need to acknowledge *effort* rather than cleverness, *personality* rather than appearance, learning *style* rather than the outcome.

Specific feedback should thus focus on the *process* that the children use or dispositions they have exercised to achieve a final product or outcome. (Various dispositions were listed in Chapter 3.) You might comment on the effort children have expended: 'Looks like you planned how to go about that before starting it' or, when they have shared with a playmate: 'I appreciate that you thought of Tia and gave her a turn'.

If you would like to supplement this everyday feedback with a formal activity, you could make a list with vulnerable children of all the things they can achieve. In making the list, you can write down *anything* that they have ever done: a single instance is enough to tell you that they can do it, even if they do not do it all the time. Don't qualify these statements with 'sometimes' or 'when he tries' or with descriptions of how well they perform activity: if they insist that you write down that, for example, they can run fast, you make that two items: 'Jake can run' and, 'Jake can run fast'.

Teach children to evaluate negative feedback. At times, everyone will fail at something and will be snubbed or rejected by other people. It is important that individuals notice this sort of negative feedback about themselves, especially when it is valid. But it is also important not to let a single failure define ourselves as failures in general, or take other people's opinions of us more seriously than we take our own (Katz 1995).

So, when they are disappointed in themselves, your first response to children is to listen and accept what they feel. They will think that you do not understand them if you insist on reassuring them that things aren't that bad, or if you tell them to cheer up. (Chapter 7 details that reassuring others blocks communication with them.)

If children are reacting to invalid criticism or are expecting unrealistically high performances from themselves, you might gently ask whether they are being realistic, without giving advice or telling them off for feeling what they feel. You could, for example, ask gently, 'You seem disappointed that it is hard for you to build that. But do you think you can build with blocks like a three year old? Isn't that all you can expect when you're still three?'

But also realise that children's self-esteem will fluctuate from time to time. An occasional low period is not a cause for alarm.

Satisfy children's needs. As already mentioned, young children describe themselves by how they look, what they wear, how healthy they are, and what they own. You could suggest to parents that they help their children to value themselves by meeting their needs in these areas. For example, the children could be given some choice about their haircut and clothes, so that they like and feel good about their appearance (without being obsessed with it). Parents can get help if their children have a health condition, so that the children feel in control of their own bodies and what happens to them. And parents might give their children permission not to share some special toys, so that the children have at least one possession that they can call their own.

Facilitate children's friendships. Friendships not only meet children's social needs but also feed their self-esteem. From the feedback that children receive from their friends, they learn about who they are. Therefore, give children plenty of opportunities to play with their peers. If they have trouble entering a group because of shyness or lack the confidence to be assertive with playmates, help them to learn to overcome these difficulties (see Chapter 5).

Encourage realistic ideals

As we have seen so far, self-esteem is the measure of how well we achieve the standards we expect of ourselves. As well as making children more aware of the things they *can* do—that is, expanding their self-concept—you can also help them to set realistic expectations for themselves.

Accept yourself. Children copy how we adults handle our own achievements and failures. If we accept ourselves—even our own mistakes—surrounding children will learn from us how to be gentle with themselves too. So when you make a mistake, do not put yourself down. If you talk to yourself harshly, onlooking children will learn to do the same to themselves. Even if you console *them* when they are disappointed in themselves, they will not be convinced by what you say about their mistakes but will copy what you *do* about your own.

Sometimes it might be useful to say positive things about yourself in children's hearing, so that they learn how to acknowledge their own successes. You might comment positively: 'I've been really organised today' or, 'I'm a star!' or, 'One thing I like about me is . . .' or, 'I'm really good at . . .' or, 'I'm pleased I chose that book to read. You all seemed to enjoy it'.

Prohibit put-downs. Adults often talk about children in ways that put them down, even when we do not mean to. Sometimes, we do so when disciplining them when, instead of giving a simple command, we add a comment such as: 'Give that back. That's very selfish'. Negative labels or disparaging nicknames for children can become self-fulfilling—or like seeds in children's minds—that grow into a negative self-concept (Biddulph 1993).

We might also incite children to fail by giving instructions that tell them what *not* to do ('Don't fall') instead of what they could do: 'Watch your feet carefully'. Or we encourage behaviour that will limit them in the long run. For example, we might tell children that being shy is 'cute', or comment in their hearing that they are not very good at a particular task.

Using *emotional blackmail* to get children to behave will also lower their self-esteem. One form of this is *using guilt to control children*: 'You make me sad when you do that'. Sometimes, such negative messages are reinforced by *ridicule* if children challenge the implied negative opinion of them: 'You can't take a joke, can you?' . . . 'Don't be silly. I didn't mean it.' . . . 'Grow up, don't be a baby'. In fact, children *never* have a sense of humour about being put down, because it isn't funny.

Finally, we adults have copied some habits that devalue children such as forgetting to introduce them when we are introducing adults; speaking about children in front of them as if they cannot hear or don't care what we are saying; or denying them things they want because their wishes seem silly to us. Although we do not usually intend to cause hurt by such carelessness, these actions inadvertently tell children that we do not value them.

Avoid comparison and competition. Children will develop low self-esteem if we compare them to someone who is more capable than them. Our feedback, therefore, must comment only on the processes each child uses, not on the differing quality of their outcomes.

Encourage risk-taking. If being successful makes children 'good' boys and girls, they will assume that making a mistake renders them 'bad' and so they will restrict themselves to only the safest of activities to avoid failure. One of the many advantages, then, of acknowledgment is that it gives children permission to be adventurous and risk getting things wrong. This will advance their learning.

Accept mistakes. Children will become discouraged if we expect them to get things right every time or to 'do their best' always. When we point out their errors, they might learn that making mistakes is wrong, when instead if they are not making mistakes, that means they already knew how to do a task. This is not called learning: it is *practising*. So, when children have not been as successful as you or they would have hoped, it is still important to comment on what they *did* achieve.

You can also teach children to live by the following maxims:

Self-affirming statements

Strive for excellence, not perfection.

On worthwhile tasks, strive to *do* your best, not to *be* the best.

Have the courage to be imperfect.

Don't let failure go to your head.

If you wanted, you could actually teach children how to make deliberate mistakes by doing something together and failing at it badly. You might bake a horrible cake or try to lose at a game. The only rule is that deliberate mistakes must be safe so that no-one is hurt.

A make-a-mistake game can be fun too. One caregiver can be the coach who plots with the children what mistake they will make today, while the other adult has to try to guess what it was. If the other caregiver 'cannot' guess what the mistake was, she has to give the child a special treat or do something silly. Meanwhile of course, behind the scenes, the colleagues are plotting all this together.

Accepting mistakes refers not just to the times when children make developmental errors—when they cannot complete a puzzle or when they write their letters backwards, or whatever—but to behavioural mistakes too. Children will not profit from the mixed message to be adventurous and creative when learning but to conform and do as they are told when behaving (McCaslin & Good 1992). So you will need to accept that mistakes in both domains—learning and behaviour—are inevitable, and are an occasion for teaching and learning more skills, rather than a trigger for punishment.

Conclusion

Young babies get very excited when they walk for the first time, which shows that they already know how to notice when they are successful. At the other end of the age range, we adults need to evaluate our own efforts, because none of us would want to be holding our breath waiting for someone else to tell us that we're wonderful. But in between, we train children out of noticing when they do well.

Yet self-esteem is literally that: *self*-evaluation. Children might doubt other people's opinions of them, but they will believe their own. Therefore, we need to teach children how to assess their own actions and how to set realistic standards for themselves. Being able to do this will directly help their self-esteem throughout life. As well, children who can monitor their successes have learnt also how to notice their behaviour—and so it is only a small step to learn how to notice when their behaviour might harm someone else. This is the basis of learning to behave considerately.

Suggested further reading

Many children's books have themes about self-esteem; for your own reading I recommend:

Berne, P.H. & Savary, L.M. (1996). *Building self-esteem in children.* (exp. ed.) New York: Crossroad Publishing.

Biddulph, S. (1993). *The secret of happy children.* (rev ed.) Sydney: Bay Books/ Minneapolis, MN: Free Spirit.

Curry, N.E. & Johnson, C.N. (1990). *Beyond self-esteem: Developing a genuine sense of human value.* Washington, DC: National Association for the Education of Young Children.

Seligman, M.E.P. (1995). *The optimistic child.* Sydney: Random House.

5

● ●

Meeting children's social needs

> *A community is a group of individuals who have a serious stake in each other's well-being and who can accomplish together that which they could not do alone . . . Practices that ignore the reality of children's deep need for a sense of community are educationally unsound.*
>
> KATZ AND MCCLELLAN (1997: 17)

The quality of the interactions between staff and children and among the children will affect the overall quality of the care that the children experience at the time and will promote the children's developmental skills, both in the short and long terms (Doherty-Derkowski 1995). This is clearly sufficient reason to meet children's social needs. But given the topic of this book, there is also a behaviour management rationale that if you relate to children with acceptance and warmth, they will come to care about you and so are more likely to consider your needs and value your good opinion of their behaviour; and children who know and care about their peers are less likely to act unkindly towards them.

Connectedness to adults

Behaviour management is to be based on protective, nurturing, encouraging and educational relationships between you and the children in your care (Rodd 1996). The first cornerstone of this relationship is trust. This develops when children are able to anticipate what is going to happen to them

(Gerber 1981). When adults are cued into and listen to children's needs, the children in turn learn to trust their caregivers and develop confidence in the quality and consistency of their caring.

Continuity of care

As long as individual caregivers are not burdened, every attempt needs to be made to ensure continuity of adult care of each child (Elicker & Fortner-Wood 1995). This is especially necessary for children with disturbed or stressed attachments to their parents and those whose behaviour is troublesome.

Attachment

Attachment refers to babies' emotional ties with adults; bonding refers to adults' affection for the baby (Klass 1999). Unlike in other species (for example, ducklings and lambs) in which attachment is instantaneous (where it is termed imprinting), human babies take many months to develop attachment to their parents. (We know that it is complete when infants develop 'stranger anxiety' at around 6–8 months of age.)

Babies attach to those who are sensitive to how they are feeling and who respond appropriately to what they need. It does not have to do with how much time the carer and baby spend together. (This assertion is supported by the fact that infants attach to their father, even if he spends very little time with them.) When others are sensitive to them and supply what they need, babies can predict and control their environment.

For babies to develop a strong attachment to you, they need you to respond to them in the following ways (Peterson 1996: 156–157).

- They need frequent affectionate contact with you.
- They need timely assistance when distressed—that is, for you to notice that they are upset.
- They need appropriate help to alleviate their distress—that is, they need you to be sensitive to what is causing their discomfort and to provide what may help.
- They need you to talk to them when they are being vocal.
- They need you to stimulate their thinking through play.

When children are confident that they will be looked after, they tend to explore their environment more, persist with solving problems, and be interested in learning. As a result, their thinking and social skills are enhanced and they are more likely as adults to be comfortable with intimate relationships (Peterson 1996).

And in terms of the topic of this book—disciplinary approaches—it is clear that when you respond to children's needs, they are more likely in return to want to cooperate with what you need. They will care about you—because you care about them—and so will want to please you.

Accept children

A study of preschool children's compliance with teachers' directives found that children followed directives 100% of the time when teachers' approval rates were high, and only 14% when teachers' approval was low (Atwater & Morris 1988). This, then, supports the notion that children are willing to accede to requests when their teachers are responsive to them.

Thus, while we must keep in mind that the main purpose of fostering warm relationships between caregivers and children is for the emotional support and nurturance that this offers children, in the context of this book's focus on behaviour management practices, caregivers' acceptance of children is likely to increase children's willingness to cooperate with adults' directives.

Acceptance entails accepting the diversity of children's interests, backgrounds, activity levels and behaviour. It also means accepting their feelings. Fields and Boesser (2002) make the point that some adults believe that 'little people have little feelings' when in fact children's emotions are as meaningful to them as ours are to us. So it is important that you accept what they are feeling even if you do not understand why they feel in a given way.

Relate warmly with children

Your relationship with children needs to involve attention, acceptance, appreciation, affirmation and affection (Albert 1989, in Rodd 1996). With respect to the first of these qualities, it has been found that although educators spend the vast majority of their time interacting with children, nearly one-third of the children actually receive no individual attention on a given day, which signals the need for adults consciously to make contact with individual children who otherwise could be overlooked (Kontos & Wilcox-Herzog 1997).

With respect to the remaining qualities, your interactions with children must be warm and fun and offer opportunities for personal two-way discussions in which you listen to what interests them, rather than asking questions whose answers you already know (such as, 'What colour are you using now?') or giving directives (NCAC 1993). It is important that both what you say and how you say it conveys respect for children; accepts their individuality and promotes their autonomy; supports their social learning; and is responsive to their needs.

In short, you need to be sensitive and responsive to children's current needs. This involves reacting appropriately and promptly to their signals, listening to children with attention and respect, initiating activities that reflect the children's developmental level and interests, and being sensitive to the children's current mood and situation (Doherty-Derkowski 1995). These behaviours tell children that they 'are cared *about* as well as cared for' (Doherty-Derkowski 1995: 36).

Listen

Chapter 7 discusses the importance of listening to children, so that information will not be repeated here. Suffice it to say now that not only must we listen to what children say, but also to what their behaviour is communicating about their needs. Today's uncooperative behaviour can look as if it is just naughty or obstinate or obstructive, but it is useful at difficult times to remember that their behaviour is the only way that young children can convey that they are not coping. In that case, we must read these signs.

Use a guidance approach to behavioural disruptions

Dealing with challenging behaviour is actually not about you and it is not about individual children: it has to do with your *relationship*. Think about how you would feel about your supervisor if he or she told you off for a mistake that you had made on the job. Now imagine how you would feel if the chastisement occurred in front of your colleagues. It is a safe bet that you would not feel warmly towards your supervisor: you certainly would not be inclined to invite him or her out for a meal to cement your relationship!

So it is with children. When we attempt to correct their behaviour using the controlling approaches of rewards and punishments, they are subsequently less—not more—likely to want to have anything to do with us. As a result, not only have we severed a potential source of nurturing for the children, we have destroyed the only currency we have for correcting their behaviour: they will not value our good opinion of them so will be less concerned if they disappoint us.

When instead you have built up a history with children of listening to them and accommodating their objections when possible and reasonable, you will find that the children want to be similarly considerate of you. When you have cooperated with their individual needs, they will be willing to cooperate with yours. The genuine affection that you share will enhance your lives and—with respect to the focus of this book—will give you a strong foundation from which to guide their behaviour.

Friendships

Friendship is an ongoing, voluntary bond between individuals who see themselves as roughly equal, have a mutual preference for each other, share emotional warmth and interact reciprocally (Hartup 1989; Howes 1983a). It usually requires that the children are at a similar developmental level and behave predictably so that others feel safe in their company.

Friendships are fundamental to children's satisfaction with their care or preschool experience (Langsted 1994, in Pugh & Selleck 1996). They can be facilitated naturally in a supportive setting where the peer group is stable and the caregivers familiar (Lady Gowrie Child Centre Melbourne 1987). However, for some children, friendships might not necessarily develop naturally and so these isolated youngsters will need your help to find companionship.

Socially isolated children

Three groups of children are more likely than most to be socially isolated in early childhood centres. First is children with significant intellectual delays: around 30% are actively rejected—which is often related to their behavioural difficulties—while a greater number still are ignored (or neglected) by peers, which is often related to their social reticence and less sophisticated social skills (Odom et al. 1999).

A second group of potentially isolated children are those with advanced development. Gifted youngsters are often popular with others but do not experience these relationships as deeply companionable: in short, many are not as attached to peers as their peers are to them. They might develop deep attachments to a best friend at a similar developmental level to themselves or to their parents—but lack a breadth of attachments, making them vulnerable to separation problems and loneliness within groups of age mates. Thus, despite the fact that their advanced problem-solving skills contribute to social finesse, it can seem at times that they lack the ability to form friendships. The main intervention for these children is to give them access to others at their developmental level, as usually their social success improves and they feel less lonely when they have playmates who can share their sophisticated interests.

A third group of children commonly experiencing social isolation are those who frequently behave aggressively. Although these children initially approach others often, their overtures are frequently rejected because their approaches are often boisterous or aggressive, they disrupt others' play and are less cooperative—with the result that over time they initiate less often and become increasingly isolated (Dodge 1983). As a result of their behaviour, these children are often disliked by many peers but are liked by and gravitate towards other aggressive children (Arnold et al. 1999; Dodge 1983; Farver 1996; Hartup 1989; Hartup & Moore 1990).

Social skills interventions

Although you cannot impose friendships on children, you can create the conditions in which friendships may flourish. Once isolated, children's social inclusion is unlikely to improve without deliberate intervention: it is not enough simply to place children together and hope that they will relate to each other positively (Guralnick et al. 1998). This is especially true when individual children behave aggressively to their peers, as that naturally is likely to lead to social rejection.

Promote acceptance

When children observe you interacting positively with all children, they are likely to accept and involve otherwise neglected children in their play (Okagaki et al. 1998). As well as in your everyday interactions, your acceptance can be communicated by talking openly with the group about the many differences and similarities between people so that those who are isolated for reasons of appearance or ability levels can be seen to be similar to—and thus potential companions for—surrounding children (Crary 1992).

Ensure that the children know each other

Children are more willing to play with someone whom they know. This requires that, where possible, you maintain a stable group membership and on a daily basis incorporate the likes of name songs in your group story and song sessions so that the children become familiar with each other.

Consider placement

Because children choose playmates who are at their own developmental level, it behoves us to provide individual children with potential matches by, where possible, placing children with disabilities with at least one other child with a similar disability (Freeman & Kasari 1998)—and gifted children with older playmates—so that they have access to peers at similar developmental levels to themselves (see Chapters 3 and 13).

Provide toys that invite social play

Ensure that the activities on offer invite social play and are more attractive than being alone. Toys that tend to invite isolated or parallel play include small building blocks, playdough, books, sand play, computer games, and craft activities; while those that promote social cooperative play comprise the likes of dress-up clothes, dolls and doll houses, large blocks, housekeeping materials and vehicles (Ivory & McCollum 1999). However, this list is not prescriptive as most of the social category of toys can be used in solitary play as well, while the provision of dramatic play equipment (such as kitchen utensils with playdough) will allow children to engage cooperatively with otherwise solitary materials (Sainato & Carta 1992).

Initiate cooperative activities

You can actively foster cooperative play between children by instigating activities and games that require joint effort and cooperation. Cooperative games aim to involve isolated children and to pair up children who ordinarily do not play with each other. In this way, they expand each child's pool of potential friends; help children to form a cohesive group; teach cooperation skills, turn-taking and sharing; decrease aggressiveness; and provide a non-threatening context for modelling and rehearsing social skills (Bay-Hinitz et al. 1994; Hill & Reed 1989; Orlick 1982; Sapon-Shevin 1986; Swetnam et al. 1983).

Examples of cooperative games include non-elimination musical chairs which involves removing a chair—not a player—whenever the music stops, so that all the children end up having to fit on the one remaining chair. Another example is the frozen bean bag game that requires children to move around with a small bean bag on their heads, freezing when it falls off and remaining still until another child helps by replacing the bean bag on their head (Sapon-Shevin 1986).

At the same time, you must curb competitive activities, as these increase aggressive behaviours and reduce cooperation (Bay-Hinitz et al. 1994). Competitive games involve taunting or teasing (such as 'king of the castle'); grabbing or snatching at scarce toys (as in 'musical chairs'); monopolising or excluding other children (for instance, the 'piggy in the middle' game); or the use of physical force (such as tag ball) (Orlick 1982; Sapon-Shevin 1986).

Some children are reluctant at first to engage in cooperative games but nevertheless still benefit from even low participation rates and can be persuaded to participate by watching the other children enjoying themselves (Bay-Hinitz et al. 1994; Hill & Reed 1989).

Provide some solitude

Around one-quarter of children can be expected to prefer their own company to being surrounded by numerous other individuals. For these introverted children and all those who occasionally seek some solitude, provide a quiet corner to which they can retreat. Being allowed to withdraw can encourage children's participation when they are ready and can avoid behavioural outbursts that are provoked by feeling crowded.

Mediate children's use of social skills

When you observe that particular children have no stable friendships, are rejected because of their aggressive behaviour, have disabilities that impair their social skilfulness, or play predominantly alone or in parallel beyond the usual age, you can take active steps to support their social engagement.

In most instances, it is important to allow children to direct their own play and resolve their nonviolent conflicts independently (Harrison & Tegel 1999). However, when children are chronically isolated, you can be more directive by:

- selecting socially competent children to play alongside a reticent child;
- introducing an activity that will attract that child and others; and
- if necessary, prompting their play until the children can direct it themselves (Odom et al. 1999).

Teach specific behaviours that make up social skilfulness

The first social skill is surveillance: to enter a group, children need to take time to survey the group's activities and members' non-verbal behaviours. This allows hopeful entrants to make their behaviour congruent with the group's, which in turn makes it more likely that their bids to gain entry will be positively received (Asher 1983; Brown et al. 2000). A hopeful entrant can then approach the other children and wait for a natural break to occur and then begin to do what the other children are doing (Putallaz & Wasserman 1990). This has been called the wait-and-hover technique and is extremely useful—as long as it is followed by bids to enter; otherwise children remain on the periphery for extended periods (Brown et al. 2000).

This entry process can be facilitated by the use of some social behaviours, as listed in Box 5.1. You can naturalistically prompt and assist isolated children to use any of these behaviours. Then, once children have located some playmates, they need to know how to maintain the relationship. This too requires a range skills as outlined in Box 5.1.

Box 5.1: Prosocial skills

Although social skills differ at various ages and for various ethnic and cultural groups, some skills are universal. These universal skills comprise being positive and agreeable; being able to use relevant contextual and social cues to guide one's own behaviour; and being sensitive and responsive to the interests and behaviour of playmates (Mize 1995).

Entry skills

In order for children to be successful in their bids to enter a group, they need to be competent at employing the following range of entry skills.

- **Observation** of a group before attempting entry.
- **Use of initiations** such as: approaching, touching, gaining eye contact, vocalising or using another child's name.
- **Positive responses to others' invitations**.
- **Avoidance of disruptive actions,** such as calling attention to oneself, asking questions, criticising the way the other children are playing, introducing new topics of conversation or new games, being too boisterous and thus out of keeping with the group, acting aggressively, or destroying others' play materials (Putallaz & Gottman 1981; Putallaz & Wasserman 1990).

Supportive actions

Having gained entry to the play of others, the playmates need to be able to sustain their interaction. This will require the use of the following social skills.

- **Use of supportive behaviours.** These tell others that one is keen to cooperate and can be trusted. Such actions comprise: complimenting, smiling at, cooperating with, imitating, sharing, taking turns and assisting others in play.
- **Diplomatic leads.** Children need to be able to make positive play suggestions to enlist other children in their play without being bossy.
- **Seek support.** Children need to be able to ask questions or seek assistance from their playmates. Sometimes, requests can be framed as questions so that they seem less directive.

(Continued)

Box 5.1: *(Continued)*

- **Comment on play.** Statements serve to remind the players of their play theme, establish common ground, and help the children to function cohesively (Mize 1995). One child might say, 'We're doing this together, aren't we?'—as a way to establish common ground with playmates and to elicit a response from them. To be effective and well received, these comments have to be relevant to and in tune with the other children.
- **Awareness of others.** Children need to pay attention to relevant social cues so that they are sensitive to the needs of their playmates. In response to feedback from their peers, they need to be able to moderate their behaviour to suit their friends and respond positively when others are trying to make friends.
- **Self-awareness.** Children need to be aware of how their behaviour will influence other people's responses to them.

Conflict management skills

To resolve conflict peaceably with playmates—such as when their requests to enter a group are being rebuffed—children need to:

- be persuasive and assertive rather than bossy;
- negotiate play activities;
- obey social rules about sharing and taking turns as leader, for example;
- suggest compromises when someone's actions have been disputed; and
- not accede to unreasonable demands from playmates but nevertheless decline tactfully by presenting a rationale for not accepting a playmate's idea or by offering an alternative suggestion (Trawick-Smith 1988).

Assist children's development

Children need to be competent at language so that they understand the play themes of others and can sustain and elaborate on their social play (Rose 1983; Rubin 1980; Trawick-Smith 1988). Similarly, they need the requisite motor skills to participate in peers' physical play. Therefore, if children speak a language other than English or have delayed skills in any developmental domain, secure them specialist assistance to improve their skills so that, in turn, their social inclusion is likely to be enhanced.

Assist peers to engage excluded children

When children are neglected or ignored by their peers, you might deliberately structure an activity that you know will appeal to two children who do not ordinarily play together, or you could await a natural opportunity to point out to a competent child that an isolated child appears interested in what he or she is doing and might want to take part. You could say something like 'James seems interested in your game. Do you think he could help you with the baby's bed?'.

A second instance when you can support individual children is when they are refused entry to other children's play, which is common even when children request entry in socially graceful ways. At times, a rebuff can occur because the children just want to be alone or because they cannot think of a way of involving a new player. In the latter case, you can inquire about their game and ask whether there is room for one more child. This approach is expanded in Chapter 12.

Provide formal coaching

When children appear to lack information about how to behave in prosocial ways, individual training sessions can prove effective. However, social skills coaching might not be effective for those aggressive children who know how to behave prosocially but who use their aggression strategically and with great success. These children will not be motivated to act more prosocially and instead will need some behaviour management to gain control of their impulses. Once their behaviour is under control, they might be able to acquire the normal social skills naturally, without structured coaching.

Training methods generally comprise teaching children about social goals such as having fun together; giving them opportunities to practise new social skills; and supplying feedback (Ladd & Mize 1983; Mize 1995; Rose 1983). An example of a program for early childhood is provided by Mize (1995). She withdrew a pair of children—one a target child who had social skill deficits and the other a popular child. She began the first coaching session by using a hand puppet to ask the children if they could help it to teach two other puppets how to have fun when they played together. The coach would act out these suggestions and then the children would rehearse them by working first the puppets and then other supplied toys themselves. During their play, the coach would use the first puppet to offer suggestions, encouragement and feedback to the children.

Over the course of the training—of around ten sessions—rehearsals became more realistic and addressed the specific skill deficits of targeted children. Finally, once they could display the skills confidently and with poise in the coaching session, prompts from adults were used to guide them in using those skills during natural play sessions at the centre (Mize 1995).

Mize's program focused on the following three key components of social competence: knowledge, skills, and self-assessment.

- **Knowledge** of the universal social skills as listed in Box 5.1 and of specific goals such as how children can have fun playing together. Mize (1995) found that trying to teach abstract concepts such as cooperating or being 'nice' was too vague for the children to comprehend.
- **Skills**. Mize focused on entry, sustaining and conflict resolution skills as listed in Box 5.1, teaching those that seemed relevant for each child.
- **Self-monitoring and self-evaluation**. The third aspect of Mize's program involved coaching children to notice other people's reactions to their behaviour, to interpret these reactions constructively, and adjust their actions accordingly.

Although young children can learn social skills quickly from coaching sessions and can learn to enact those skills in natural settings, it can take some time for the other children to respond more positively to them (Mize 1995). In the meantime, you will need to continue to offer encouragement and to structure the group—through cooperative play and the other interventions already mentioned—so that the atmosphere in the group is one of acceptance and inclusion. This will give all children—but particularly previously rejected children—the confidence to re-enter the group and will provide a safe context for making the occasional social mistake.

Conclusion

Peers can make unique contributions to children's development in many domains (see Hartup 1989; Hartup & Moore 1990), such that when children's peer relationships are disrupted, their development as well as their emotional wellbeing can suffer. In their despair, they might act in antisocial ways.

Alternatively, social isolation can arise from a lack of emotional regulation—that is, from behavioural difficulties. This, then, is not a lack of knowledge about how to behave prosocially, but a lack of self-control in social situations. In that case, a guidance approach can be used to teach children to remain in command of themselves, in ways recommended in Part 3. The resulting improvement in their behaviour will allow them to find acceptance and companionship within their peer group.

Suggested further reading

Katz, L.G. & McClellan, D.E. (1997). *Fostering children's social competence: The teacher's role*. Washington, DC: National Association for the Education of Young Children.

Kostelnick, M.J., Stein, L.C., Whiren, A.P. & Soderman, A.K. (1998). *Guiding children's social development*. (3rd ed.) Albany, NY: Delmar.

Odom, S.L., McConnell, S.R. & McEvoy, M.A. (Eds.) (1992). *Social competence of young children with disabilities: Issues and strategies for intervention*. Baltimore, MD: Paul H. Brookes.

Sapon-Shevin, M. (1999). *Because we can change the world: A practical guide to building cooperative, inclusive classroom communities*. Boston, MA: Allyn and Bacon.

Part Three

● ●

Responding to inconsiderate behaviour

The process of acquiring a set of rules, values, and, ultimately, principles, as well as using such standards as guides for behavior, takes place over the entire course of childhood and adolescence.

SROUFE (1996: 197, IN GOWEN & NEGRIB 2002: 191)

Part 3 recommends some ways for guiding children when they are behaving inconsiderately. The guidance approach accepts that children have rights but that other people do not have to suffer children's inconsiderate behaviour. It also accepts that making behavioural mistakes is a natural part of learning so, although we must teach children more thoughtful behaviours, there is no need to punish them for their mistakes.

The chapters in this part define inconsiderate behaviour as any act that interferes with someone's rights. However, this broad definition needs some further refinement. Thoughtless behaviour can come in two forms: the original incident—which Bill Rogers (1998) calls the primary behaviour—and children's reaction to being corrected—which is the secondary behaviour.

I have observed that young children often display a sequence of wrong-doings. Rather like a bee pollinating flowers, on certain days, individual children can move from one activity to another, from one group of children to another, creating havoc at each location. I once thought that these children were on the wind-up and that they were getting out of control of themselves. I still believe that this is true to some extent, but I now think that the 'wind-up' can sometimes be the result not so much of the children's feelings getting out of hand, but is a reaction to how the first incident was handled. If children feel shamed or upset by the adult's reaction to the first incident, they are much more likely to repeat another disruptive behaviour (Porter 1999b).

This means that how we respond to children's original behaviour is crucial. It makes sense to respond compassionately when they behave inconsiderately so that you do not make your job any harder by provoking another incident that requires an intervention.

We cannot expect children who are four years old to behave like they are 20, nor even to behave like they are five. But when children do not know a more mature behaviour, we should not passively accept this and hope that they will 'grow out of it': instead, we must set about teaching them what they need to know. In most cases, in the early childhood years, this does not mean repeating information about how they should be acting, but helping children develop the self-control that is necessary for them to act on the knowledge that they already possess. At those times when they lack this self-control, the intention of the guidance approach is to help them regain it, not to punish them for behaving emotionally—that is, for behaving like children.

6

○ ○

Origins of inconsiderate behaviour

> *Mistaken behavior is a natural occurrence, the result of attempts by inexperienced, developmentally young children to interact with a complicated, increasingly impersonal world.*

> GARTRELL (1998: 40)

In this chapter, I follow Rogers' (1998) distinction between primary and secondary sources of inconsiderate behaviour. Primary behaviours arise as a result of what is going on inside young children; secondary behaviours are children's reaction to correction of these primary behaviours.

Primary causes

Children's thoughtless behaviour can arise from sources within them. Their resulting disruptive acts are generally thought to be a problem because they violate the rights of the children who are performing them or interfere with the rights or needs of surrounding people.

Normal exuberance

Children will occasionally become elated and excited about simply being alive and will engage in rowdy behaviour that unintentionally inconveniences or irritates surrounding individuals.

Normal exploration

It is natural—and essential—that children explore their social world, just as they do their physical world. This will inevitably result in mistakes because children are too young always to be able to anticipate the effect of their actions on others. Although normal, exploratory behaviours of young children can be inconvenient to adults. They might explore dangerous aspects of their environment or might test whether you are serious about a prohibition. These behaviours can be trying to busy adults, but are normal for children, and seldom violate others' rights.

Lack of skill

Children might lack the ability to perform a more mature behaviour because:

- **of their age** they have not been alive long enough to have learned how to act thoughtfully;
- **of their developmental level** some children will have a disability that impairs their learning or is associated with abnormal behaviours—such as head-banging and biting oneself—that are aberrant at any age (Smith et al. 1987);
- **they have a disorganised nervous system**. When children have particular disabilities such as autism, sensory integration difficulties (see Soden 2002a or 2002b), or (perhaps) ADHD, were exposed in utero to drugs or neurotoxins, or have food intolerances, their behaviour can become irregular as a result of disturbed information processing by their nervous system;
- **they are copying inappropriate role models** such as when children who are raised aggressively become violent with their playmates, as this is the only means that they have learned for solving disputes.

Skill deficits come with the territory and become an issue only if the children are of an age to know how to act more considerately but are not doing so. We all realise that under-two-year-olds do not have the skills to behave maturely and so we excuse their ineptness. However, beyond that age we start to expect more skilful behaviour. Nevertheless, older children might know the suitable skill to use, but are out of control of themselves and so cannot use it. This, then, is the fourth type of primary behavioural difficulty.

Loss of self-control

Young children can become disorganised very easily. If they are tired, hungry, or stressed, they feel overwhelmed and cannot organise themselves to use a skill that at other times they can display: even when they know what to do, they cannot do it. Temporarily, they do not have sufficient command of themselves to be able to use their skills appropriately. Their feelings get out of control and they lose the plot. For example, they might not use words to ask a playmate for a toy, but will snatch it because they want it *now*.

It is normal and quite common for young children's feelings to get out of balance, because babies have to act on every feeling and communicate what they need, so that they receive the care they require to stay alive. But adults have learned that there are times and places where acting on our feelings is not suitable. It takes us the 16 or so years of childhood to move from our baby state to our adult state, and so we cannot expect young children to have mastered their feelings already.

It is even normal for adults sometimes to lack self-control. When we are, say, trying to restrict our intake of fatty foods but are tempted to eat something that we know to be fatty, it is not a lack of information that causes us to consume the item, but a lack of self-control.

A loss of self-control is communicated by young children in the form of 'tantrums'. These are described below. They usually result in:

- **excessive behaviour**: behaviours that are normal but which occur past the usual age or at a higher rate than usual (Herbert 1987);
- **mistimed behaviours**: acts that are suitable in one time and place—such as moving about—but which disrupt the present context, such as group story time (Apter 1982, in Conway 1998).

The four 'tantrum' patterns

I have observed four patterns of behaviour which signal that children's emotions are overwhelming them. I call these patterns *tantrums*, for want of a better word, although in a way it is an unfortunate term because it could imply that the children are being deliberately obstructive. But I use it only as a shorthand way of saying that the children have become disorganised or overwhelmed and so cannot get on with the job at hand. Tantrums come in two styles: the active sort that are reasonably apparent to anyone; and the passive type which are less obvious and thus sometimes more confusing to deal with. Despite the outward differences, however, they both signal the same loss of emotional control and can be responded to in very similar ways.

The first active tantrum is the *protesting* tantrum that we have all seen— or experienced—in a shopping centre when children are angry about not getting what they want. This type of tantrum involves crying, screaming, hitting or kicking, and is very active. However, it is not very common after the age of three or so, because adults recognise it for what it is and generally deal with it successfully.

By the way, this protesting tantrum is different from pre-verbal children's attempt to communicate that they are disappointed. *That* is not a tantrum: it is legitimate communication. A tantrum is where children who can usually say what they need, instead get so worked up that they cannot use words.

A second active tantrum is *social*. This involves verbal abuse, refusing to share or take turns, bullying, name-calling, and generally not being friendly. Children having a social tantrum might have become angry with their playmate and cannot overcome this feeling to play sociably, despite knowing how to do so. Sometimes during play, two playmates have both lost control of their feelings in this way, and so both can be said to be having a social tantrum. Children can also display social tantrums towards adults.

Then there are the passive versions. First is the behaviour that tends to replace protesting tantrums—namely *whingeing*, (whining in U.S. terms), sulking or nagging. These behaviours tell us that children feel dissatisfied with something, and cannot get past that feeling to get on with what needs to be done.

The fourth and most common pattern of behaviour that signals that children are not managing to overcome their feelings is *uncooperative* behaviour. They cannot do as they are asked because they do not want to— and cannot overcome their feelings about having to do it. .

I have noticed that when children often display active tantrums (the protesting or social types), they usually exhibit one of the passive types (whingeing/whining or uncooperativeness) as well. This makes it easy to deal with the more serious, active types, because you can respond to the passive tantrums before they grow into their more active equivalents and before any real harm is done.

Secondary reactions

The primary behaviours are inevitable as children will, from time to time, have needs that are not being met and so react with disruptive behaviour. However, a second class of outbursts occur in reaction to being controlled by others. Over thirty years ago, Tom Gordon (1970) called these reactions 'the three Rs' of resistance, rebellion and retaliation. He later added submission and escape as other reactions to being controlled (Gordon 1974).

In my research into behavioural guidance in child (day) care centres, I observed that these reactions constituted the most common cause of disruptions, making up approximately three-quarters of the incidents that drew caregivers' responses (Porter 1999b). However, in reply, the adults would often try to impose still more controls . . . and the children would become still more determined to seize back control of themselves, even if only through defiance. If this figure is accurate in other settings as well, it implies that caregivers' workload in responding to disruptions could be reduced numerically to one-quarter of the present rate, simply by avoiding provoking secondary reactions by the use of a guidance rather than a controlling system of discipline (Porter 1999b). Furthermore, these secondary reactions are often very extreme and so are far more difficult to respond to than primary behaviours and so add more than their numerical value to educators' workload.

Responses to the behaviour types

This categorisation of the origins of thoughtless behaviour implies some ways to respond. First, to deal with normal exuberance or exploratory behaviour, you need to understand that it is necessary for children to act in these ways. However, when the behaviour becomes excessive and starts to inconvenience others, you can be assertive about it. But, on the whole, it is how young children are, and you will need to live with it.

With *skill deficits*, you can teach children how to act considerately and explain how that skill will benefit them and other people. Thus, when they lack skills because of their age, disability or disorganised nervous systems, this is mainly an educational issue: disruptive behaviours need to be avoided through appropriate programming and the provision of extra support to compensate for the children's additional learning difficulties.

When, however, children already know how they should be acting but are too *overwhelmed* to use this knowledge, your first option is to help them to calm down so that they are able once again to use their more mature skills (see Chapter 9). This is the 'change the child' option. It might involve something as basic as putting a tired child to bed or giving a hungry child something to eat. If that fails, you will have to change your demands because the children clearly cannot cope with what they are being asked to do. This is the 'change the demands' option.

Finally, *secondary* or reactive behavioural difficulties can be avoided by guiding children through the first incident, rather than punishing them for it. Box 6.1 summarises these responses.

The attention-seeking myth

You might have noticed that in my list of the origins of disruptive behaviours I did not mention 'attention-seeking' as a cause. This is because this explanation of behaviour is not useful. First, it is applied only to children and never to adults, implying that children are particularly prone to naughtiness. Second, it seems to me that most of today's children receive even more attention than in the past, as adults generally supervise them closely to keep them safe. If this is so, how could they need still more attention? Third, if children do seem to require additional attention, this must be a legitimate need, one that we must not frustrate.

Box 6.1: Responses to children's behaviours

Behaviour type	Responses
Considerate	Accept Acknowledge
Exuberant or exploratory	Understand Be assertive if the behaviour becomes intrusive.
Skill deficits	Teach a more mature skill. Explain how the skill will be useful. Make program adjustments so that children can circumvent any learning difficulties. Provide extra support so they can learn considerate behaviour.
Emotionally overwhelmed (children have the skill but cannot use it)	Help the children to calm down. If they cannot calm down, change your demands.
Secondary reactions	Use guidance, not control

But if all these arguments do not convince you, a purely pragmatic one might. This is that, if you believe a particular behaviour to be 'attention-seeking', the suggested intervention—of ignoring it—does not work. Instead, it creates two problems. The first is that you will end up having to pay attention to the behaviour anyway because it becomes so dangerous, disruptive or intrusive that you cannot ignore it any more. By waiting, you teach children to persist with inconsiderate behaviour, and so you have done the wrong thing. But you are not supposed to pay attention to it when it starts, either—so whatever you do is wrong.

The second problem is that the children might think that you are doing nothing—or do not know what to do—and so they learn not to take you seriously when you give them directives about their behaviour.

In other words, the explanation that behaviour is attention-seeking is not useful as its suggested means of intervention does not work. Therefore, instead of believing that the children are seeking attention, it might pay to think of the behaviour as a sign that they are uncertain that, when you are busy elsewhere, nevertheless you will insist that they act considerately. Because you cannot do two things at once—you cannot finish one task and manage their behaviour at the same time—you will need to become single-minded and give disruptive behaviour your full attention, in the process clarifying how you require the children to act.

Many of us do not think to do this because we think it means that the children will have 'won' and have got the attention that they were looking for. However, when you do interrupt what you are doing and clarify what you expect of children, their behaviour improves. They did not need your attention: they just were not clear that you would insist on considerate behaviour, even when you were busy.

Conclusion

The main message of this chapter is that many of the behaviours that we regard as being in need of controlling—those that Gordon (1970) called the three Rs (resistance, rebellion and retaliation)—are actually being provoked by the controlling methods that we are using to discourage them. As these types of behaviours constitute the most numerous and most serious difficulties that I observed in child (day) care centres (Porter 1999b), avoidance of them will be beneficial for the children concerned and surrounding children and adults. The chapters that follow, then, provide means for responding to the primary behaviours listed here in ways that do not provoke children into defiance against adult domination.

7

• •

Communicating to solve problems

'Real' listening requires courage, generosity and patience on our part (Mackay 1994). It requires courage, because if we seriously entertain another's ideas it makes us vulnerable as we move out of our own comfort zone and see another point of view that could challenge our own or reveal it as flawed. Listening requires our generosity, because it is something we do for another person even when the message is less than welcome or is unattractive to us. Finally, listening requires patience because we need to suspend our own thoughts, questions and judgments and make sure we have understood the message before responding to it.

PORTER AND MCKENZIE (2000: 136)

When children are telling you by their behaviour that they are stressed, you must listen to that message and act on it. Listening, then, is the single most crucial skill for solving problems. On the other hand, when their behaviour is interfering with what you or another child in your care need, you must explain the effect that their behaviour is having. You must say what you require—firmly but without hostility. The third—and most common— situation is when children's behaviour is both disrupting their own participation in the program and having deleterious effects on others. In that case, you will need to employ the collaborative problem-solving steps. All three communication tools are described in this chapter.

Listening

Listening requires that you are willing to listen rather than trying to impose your own ideas on others. It entails giving children attention, noticing their feelings as well as their words, and actively reflecting what they are saying. To do all this well, you will need to abandon the idea that you are responsible for fixing children's 'negative' feelings but instead support them to resolve these themselves.

Attention

When you want to tell children that you are interested in hearing something that is important to them, you will need to pay attention. This is hard to do when you are busy, but genuine attention means stopping everything else—and just listening.

Invitation to talk

You can invite others to talk with you by noticing what their behaviour is telling you about how they are feeling. You can listen with your eyes, and tell them what you see: 'You look a bit sad'. . .'You seem excited'. You might add: 'Do you want to tell me about it?' and then wait quietly while they decide if and how they want to talk.

Once they have begun talking, you can say very little—maybe just 'mm-hmm' 'oh' or 'really?'—or you can repeat back the last few words that they have said to encourage them to carry on. It pays to ask very few questions—especially ones that call for a yes/no answer—because questions will direct, rather than follow, what children are telling you and can make them feel that they are being subjected to an inquisition instead of being listened to.

Listen for feelings

It can be difficult for many adults to handle children's strong feelings, even positive ones such as joy or excitement. It can be especially difficult to accept when children are angry at us. People who believe in controlling children simply do not allow them to be angry at adults. But when using a guidance approach, you can reflect the feeling that caused the children's anger: 'I can see you're hurt that I didn't help you out when you wanted me to'.

Identifying young children's emotions can be difficult because they do not have a wide vocabulary to describe how they feel. For this reason, you will have to teach infants some words to describe their feelings.

Reflection

When listening to children's feelings, it can help to reflect these back to them. You can reflect the *content*, the *feeling*, or the *meaning* behind what they are telling you. You can do this by paraphrasing or summarising what they are saying. Bolton (1987: 51) describes paraphrasing as giving:

- a concise response
- stating the essence
- of the content
- in the listener's own words.

At first, reflecting back what someone is saying can seem very false—silly, almost. It sounds as if you will be saying the obvious. Or you might worry about getting it wrong. But children will not mind if you misinterpret what they are saying—as long as you are trying to understand them. And as to saying the obvious, well, reflection will help you both become clearer about the children's feelings. Try it: it works.

Box 7.1: Roadblocks to communication

Instead of genuine listening, we can easily fall into the trap of saying things that discourage others from talking to us. Gordon (1970) described twelve common conversation habits that he called 'roadblocks to communication'. The following list of these roadblocks gives examples of how each one might unwittingly be used with young children.

Judging

It is important that you accept children's feelings, even when these are different from yours. This means not judging children for feeling something ('Don't be silly: it's not that bad'). The judging roadblocks include:

- **Criticising or blaming.** These responses do not accept what children are feeling. We might, for example, tell them that they would not have got hurt if they had obeyed the rule to walk on the path. This does not communicate any empathy for their pain, which they will think is unfair.
- **Praising** children tries to talk them out of their feelings, as when we say to a child who is reluctant to eat his lunch: 'You're such a good boy, I know you will eat up properly'.

(Continued)

Box 7.1: *(Continued)*

- **Name-calling** is much the same and has similar effects to criticising and blaming children.
- **Diagnosing** or **interpreting** what children are feeling is an attempt to tell them what their 'real' problem is and ignores their view of it. 'You don't want to go outside because Melissa hit you yesterday'.

Sending solutions

Sometimes, instead of listening, we are quick to tell children what we think they should do about their problem. Giving our own solutions can take five forms:

- **Directing** children to stop what they are feeling or doing: 'I don't care what you want: you're doing this *now*.' This tells them that their needs are not important: they must do what you want, not what they want.
- **Threatening** imposes your solution on children: 'If you don't get ready *right now* for nap time, I will make you stay in bed longer'. Threats make children fearful, resentful, and liable to test you to see if you will carry out what you threaten.
- **Preaching** explains to children why they should feel differently: 'You should come and listen to the story or you won't learn enough to be ready to start school'. Preaching is patronising because it treats children as if they did not know this already.
- **Interrogating** asks a series of questions to try to get to the bottom of the problem. When a child is reluctant to stay at your centre, you might, for instance ask questions such as: 'Didn't you have a good time yesterday?' Probing suggests that you are about to find a solution for children, instead of trusting them to find their own.
- **Advising** is an attempt to impose a positive solution: 'Perhaps you can play with Alice, so that you have some company'. Although the solution is meant to be positive, it still tells children to get over their feelings before they are ready.

Giving advice is probably the most common of the roadblocks because we all want to help children to feel better. But giving advice has many disadvantages. First, it tells children that you will not listen to them because you did not wait to hear what was the real problem: if the answer were that obvious, they would have thought of it already.

(Continued)

Box 7.1: *(Continued)*

Second, giving advice tells them that you think they are not capable of finding their own solutions, and it does not give them any practice at solving their own problems. But at the same time, giving advice makes it unlikely that children will do as you suggest because it was not their idea and so you will have to supervise their observance of the solution, and they will feel resentful. All this makes your job harder than it needs to be.

Avoiding the other person's feelings

A third group of communication roadblocks tries to take the heat out of children's feelings, usually because these upset us. This class of roadblocks includes:

- **Distracting** children from their worries, without letting them resolve these. For example, in an attempt to distract them, adults often blame a 'naughty step' for causing children's fall. Sometimes, the children are in a frame of mind to enjoy the joke but if we ignore their real distress often enough, they will learn to stop talking with us about things that matter to them.
- **Logical argument** sends the message: Don't feel: Think: 'You actually like vegetables when you taste them. You know you do'.
- **Reassuring** tries to change how children are feeling, and tells them that they are not allowed to feel badly because it upsets you. Reassurance ignores the depth of children's feelings, telling them that you do not understand them. We often tell children who have hurt themselves not to cry, for example, when instead we need to acknowledge that it hurts. Only when their pain has been recognised will they be willing to hear that it will get better.

The thirteenth roadblock

Robert Bolton (1987), who wrote a handy book on communication skills, adds a thirteenth communication roadblock to Gordon's 'dirty dozen'. He says that accusing other people (blaming them) or feeling guilty ourselves for using the communication roadblocks, is itself a communication stopper.

So, rather than feeling guilty if you recognise that you use some of the communication roadblocks described here, begin translating your

(Continued)

Box 7.1: *(Continued)*

> common responses into true listening responses. You might divide a page vertically down the middle and write down on one side of your page some of the comments you hear yourself saying to children. Then, on the other side, translate these into true listening responses. (You might also find that the translations are closer to what you intended to say in the first place.) Finally, practise using the genuine listening responses in future.

Non-verbal listening

Listening tells children that you accept them. Your own non-verbal behaviours can let them know this too, when you maintain good eye contact while they are talking with you, use a courteous tone of voice with even the youngest of children, and make sure that you chat about things that interest them, instead of talking only when you want to give an instruction.

A final non-verbal message that tells children that you accept them is not interfering with what they are doing. Letting them do a task their way tells them that you believe in their abilities. Although we want children to improve their skills, they will learn more if we let them discover things for themselves than if we tell them the answer.

Assertiveness

After listening, being assertive is the second foundation stone for teaching children to consider other people. When children are violating your rights or those of surrounding children, you will need to tell them the effect their behaviour is generating. When doing so, the key difference between asserting your needs and being aggressive lies in the language you use. When we tell children about themselves—using language such as 'That's selfish' or 'You're not doing as I asked' and use the word 'you'—this is considered aggressive; when we tell children about ourselves and the effect of their behaviour on us and use the word 'I': that is assertiveness.

Types of assertive messages

Many of us have never been taught how to construct assertive messages and we are seldom told that there are two phases to their delivery: first, saying what we require and, second, *listening* to the recipient's reaction. The following formulas can help you frame the first part positively (Jakubowski & Lange 1978); the preceding discussion on listening will help you deal with others' response to your message.

'I want' statements

Sometimes when we tell others what we want, they misinterpret this as a demand instead of a request. So, it can help to qualify your statement in some way. One way to do this is to ask how willing or able the other person is to do as you ask. For instance: 'I would like a few minutes to select today's book. Can you wait for a few moments for me to do that?'.

A second way to qualify a request is to rate how strongly you would like it: 'I want you to all to sit on your bottoms so the people behind you can see. This is a number eight want' (on a scale of 1 to 10). If the children are too young to understand numbers, you could use gaps between the fingers ('this much') or between outstretched arms ('thi . . . i . . . is much') to illustrate how strongly you need something.

A third approach is to state what your request means and doesn't mean: 'I would like everyone to leave the computer and play outside for a few minutes while the sun is shining. You can come back inside once you've had a run around (letting the children know how long they will be deprived of the computer).

'I feel' statements

These are in the form of:

When you (*do such and such*)

I feel (*x*)

Because (*my rights are being violated in this way*).

The statement does not have to be this formal, although usually it will contain each element, for example: 'I get annoyed when you don't come inside when I first ask and I have to come and remind you' which in its formal version can be seen to contain the elements: 'When you *won't come when I call you*, I feel *annoyed* because *I have to come to get you*'.

We often deliver the first two parts of an 'I feel' message, and forget the 'because', leaving children to guess our reasons. But children often cannot do this, even though the reason seems obvious to us, and so it is safer to say why you require something.

Mixed feeling statements

In this assertion method, you name more than one feeling and explain why you feel each. For example:

'I appreciate that you helped by playing quietly outside when the babies were asleep this morning. I'm disappointed now, though, that you are playing your instruments outside their window and might wake them up.'

Empathic assertion

This assertive message conveys that you understand the other person, but still expresses your own needs. For instance:

'I know that you're enjoying yourself, and it's fun to run and make noise with your friends. I am worried that you will crash into the younger children, though, so I need you to find another game to play or somewhere safe to run.'

This method is the most helpful type of assertive message, as it demonstrates to children how to listen, given that you begin by listening to them. Sensitivity to their needs builds goodwill as it tells children that you are willing to listen to them and so, as we saw in Chapter 3, this makes them more willing in return to consider you.

Confrontive assertion

This is useful when children have broken an agreement about their behaviour. The confrontive assertive message has three parts:

1. You describe in a non-judgmental way what the two of you agreed to.
2. You describe what the child did.
3. Next, you say what you want to do about that.

For example:

'We agreed that you would play by yourself until you were able to share in a friendly way with Dimitri. I see that you have come back to the sandpit and taken the bucket he was using. I would like you to play somewhere else now or give Dimitri back his bucket and find a different toy to play with.'

Guidelines for sending assertive messages

Assertive messages will work best when you can follow a few simple guidelines. First, you must not blame children for how you feel: you are responsible for your feelings. If you send your 'I' message with the intent of accusing the children or making them feel guilty, it is aggressive not assertive.

Second, you will need to be accurate about the strength of your feelings, not exaggerating these as this will cause children to dismiss what you are saying, but not watering down how you feel either, as that will not impress children sufficiently that you are serious.

It is also important to name your feeling accurately. For instance, it pays not to express anger alone, because that is not the first, not the most important, thing that you feel. We usually become angry after being hurt or frightened. Saying that you were scared or hurt will be more accurate and more effective than telling children that you are angry at them.

Fourth, assertive messages should not send solutions but leave children to decide how to respond.

Finally, you will need to listen to the children's emotional reactions. They might become aggressive or defensive; they might cry, withdraw or sulk; they might complain that what you are asking is unfair; or debate the issue with you. These reactions tell you that *they* now have the problem. You will need to give them some time to digest your statement and their feelings and then use listening and reflection. For example, when children cry at a directive: 'Seems that you're too upset now to talk about it. We'll speak again later'.

Finally, repeat your assertive message. It can take from three to ten assertive messages before other people are willing to change their behaviour, so you will need to persist. And of course notice even a hint that they are willing to do as you ask, reflecting this back: 'Sounds like you'll be happy to put away the blocks. Thanks: that'll be a big help'.

Advantages of assertion

Once children can learn to consider your feedback about the effects of their behaviour on others, they benefit because they can understand what is expected of them, and surrounding individuals benefit because their rights are not being violated. Assertiveness avoids the disadvantages of non-assertion—which include a lack of respect from others, loss of self-respect, inability to control emotional outbursts that arise when adults have pushed their tolerance (patience) too far, and feeling walked over. On the other hand, it avoids the costs of aggression which are being avoided by others, loneliness, retaliation, fear, ill health, and being overwhelmed by being responsible for so much.

Collaborative problem solving

Conflict is productive in that it signals that individuals' needs are not being met. Rather than looking to blame anyone for this, we need to find a solution that allows both people to meet their needs without violating those of others.

Whether dealing with a conflict between yourself and individual children, or helping two children who are in dispute with each other, your aim will be to find a solution, not a culprit.

Guiding principle
Look for a solution not a culprit.

To resolve a dispute in a way that meets the needs of all those involved, the collaborative problem-solving process involves the following six formal steps, which in practice will usually be more fluid than described here.

1. Agree to talk it over.
2. Find out what the other person needs through listening, and tell him or her assertively—but not aggressively—what you need. This will expose where your differences lie.
3. Together, come up with ideas of what you *could* do to meet the needs of both of you. At this stage, do not evaluate how practical the suggestions are, just brainstorm all possibilities, even silly ones. If it helps, write down your ideas.
4. Next, decide which of the options you *will* do. Do not choose a compromise that doesn't meet anyone's needs, but instead persist until you find a solution that meets both your needs.
5. Decide when and how to carry out your chosen solution.
6. Once a solution is in place, check whether it is working.

Benefits and limitations of negotiation
When you negotiate with children, you are likely to arrive at a solution that is better than any of you could generate alone. The children will be more motivated to act as agreed because they participated in deciding what was to be done and you are not imposing anything on them. Therefore, you will not have to enforce the solution and the two of you can work with—not struggle against—each other. Also, helping to decide what should be done develops children's thinking skills and tells them that you think their needs are important and worthy of being considered. Although collaborating will not convince uncooperative children to consider your needs (getting them back in command of their emotions will be necessary first), the fact that you are listening to them at least invites them to listen to you in return.

Collaborative problem solving will not work when children are in danger, or when there is true time pressure to get something done. In either case, you will need to take charge without consulting with them, and explain your reasons later.

Collaboration works best when you deal with each source of irritation at the time it surfaces, rather than leaving grievances to mount up and hurt feelings to turn to anger.

Conclusion

A crucial ingredient for working with children is your own emotional self-discipline (Ginott 1972; Rogers 1998). Central to emotional discipline is that you express your feelings appropriately and do not humiliate or denigrate children through sarcasm or other means. In short, you can act spontaneously but not impulsively (Ginott 1972), practising communication skills until they become automatic and natural.

Assertiveness and collaborative problem solving work in any relationship. They are the foundation stones of finding a solution to children's inconsiderate behaviour. However, if after being told what negative effect their behaviour is having, children cannot consider your needs, this means that they are out of control of their feelings. They cannot overcome their feelings and act on what you have said. This is called a tantrum (see Chapter 6). In these cases, the children need to get back in command of themselves so that they can be responsive to the needs of those around them. The next three chapters detail ways to help them achieve this.

Suggested further reading

Bolton, R. (1987). *People skills.* Sydney: Simon and Schuster.
Faber, A. & Mazlish, E. (1999). *How to talk so kids will listen: And listen so kids will talk.* (2nd ed.) New York: Avon.
Mackay, H. (1994). *The good listener.* Sydney: Macmillan.

8

Responding to everyday disruptions

> Mistaken behavior is a natural occurrence, the result of attempts
> by inexperienced, developmentally young children to interact
> with a complicated, increasingly impersonal world. When mis-
> taken behavior occurs, adults significantly affect what children
> learn from the experience.

GARTRELL (1998: 40)

This chapter recommends some ways to respond to the everyday hassles that
arise within groups of young children. The judgment about which
approaches are effective and which unsuccessful is based on my research in
which I observed four different child (day) care centres for 200 hours in
total, recording on audiotape the interactions that arose when children's
behaviours were disrupting others. With the notable exception of
punishments, I found most of the responses solved the problem some of the
time, but that any one response could be ineffective if applied to the wrong
class of disruptions.

Graded responses

Your response has to be in tune with the seriousness of a disruption. If
particular children act thoughtlessly very occasionally, you might select one
of the first methods to be outlined here. If, however, children are repeatedly
inconveniencing their peers or adults and you have already explained to
them that this is unacceptable, the fact that this intervention is not working

suggests the need for a new response. Just as they can remember from a single instruction where the sweet biscuits are kept, so too can they remember how they should be behaving. That they are not acting as they should, then, is due to a lack of self-control, not a lack of knowledge. Continuing to educate them about the effects of their behaviour on others is pointless, as they have heard it before and it is not altering their behaviour. To follow, then, are some alternatives.

Do nothing

There are times when doing nothing is appropriate—as suggested by Graue and Walsh's (1998) self-evident statement that 'kids do stuff'. Although the 'stuff' might not always be to adults' liking, my research showed that, on occasions, inaction allowed children to continue with their play without interference until they tired of it naturally. Inaction is effective as long as what the children are doing is not harming anyone, which includes those times when they:

- are being normally exuberant;
- act in ways that might irritate you but which nevertheless harm no one—for instance, the chanting that characterises four-year-olds' experimentation with language;
- give vent to strong feelings in inoffensive ways: they might swear in frustration (rather than at someone else—see Chapter 13);
- self-correct an accidental mistake.

Inaction at these times allows 'kids to be kids' and provides them with some privacy and freedom. It gives them some space to exercise problem-solving skills independently (with follow up from you if they are not being successful, naturally) and gives them practice at negotiation.

Ignoring an established habit will not work, but with an occasional or minor disruption, it can be effective to tell children that you will not respond—that is, you will ignore it. For instance, you could tell a child who has demanded something in a sullen voice, 'Sure, I'll get that for you—once you can ask in your happy voice'. If the children are doing something irritating but not detrimental to anyone—such as when four-year-olds chant the same thing over and over again—you could say that you are ignoring them, to signal that you have noticed what they are doing and will take action if the behaviour starts to inconvenience anyone. When children are being boisterous you could signal that you are monitoring what is happening with 'I'm listening' or 'What you're doing now is fine, but please slow down near the little children so that they aren't frightened'.

On the other hand, there are at least three occasions where inaction is not wise. The first is when children leave the likes of group story time but subsequently disrupt those who remain; the second is when individual children are not managing to engage in the program; and the third is when a child is being excluded from others' play. In all of these instances, the children need active assistance, the form of which I describe below.

Defuse resistance

Sometimes, children are being uncooperative or have become sullen after making a mistake. In these cases, it might be possible to head off a full-on confrontation by helping children to cooperate, or by letting miscreants save face.

Help them to get started

We probably over-estimate young children's ability to carry out something they are told to do. It is hard for them to interrupt their train of thought or to translate a verbal instruction into action. Sometimes, they temporarily cannot overcome their distaste for an instruction they have been given. In these cases, repeating a verbal instruction is not likely to work if it hasn't already. Instead, you could move across to reluctant children and help them to get started—say, by holding their hand while they put a block into a container, or gently guiding them in the direction where they need to move.

Let children save face

As children's self-esteem is vulnerable to feelings of failure, and as discouragement can lead to further disruptions, it is important to give children a way to save face after they have made a mistake. You could say things like:

- 'Sometimes people forget to think first. You'll probably remember next time. What do you think?'
- 'Looks like that was an accident. What could you do next time so that it doesn't happen again?'
- 'I've explained that what you did was wrong. I'm sure you wouldn't have done it if you had known that. Now that you know, I expect you won't do it again.'

Because children cannot always anticipate the effects of what they do, the result can startle them enough to teach them not to do it again, and you would only humiliate them if you preached about something they already understand.

Similarly, do not force children to apologise for their mistakes. If you respond with understanding, they are likely to choose to say sorry but if they are not ready to, forcing them will not help. Perhaps in cases where two children are involved, you could tell the injured child, 'I think that Henry is sorry that he hurt you. He might be able to say so later'. (See also Chapter 12.)

Be assertive

If you are too patient or tolerant with thoughtless behaviour, the result can be that a small misdeed will grow into a really serious breach of someone's rights. Miscreants get into unnecessary trouble, develop antisocial habits, and as a result become ostracised by peers, and meanwhile you get stressed. To avoid these negative outcomes, you should assert your rights as soon as you or others are being inconvenienced by thoughtless behaviour. (See Chapter 7).

Guiding principle

Inconsiderate behaviour calls for understanding, but not patience or excuses.

When being assertive or giving instructions, do so in a tone of voice that tells children that you expect to be taken seriously. Also, make sure that your tone and your words send the same message: many adults 'flirt' with mischievous children, implying that what they are doing is amusing, but also that they should stop. This confuses children so they persist with the behaviour to clarify which message you mean.

It will also be important to frame directives in positive terms, telling children what *to* do, rather than what *not* to do. For example, if they are walking on wet floor tiles, a negative instruction would tell them not to run. But because of the way the human brain works, they will remember the word 'run' and forget the words 'do not', with the result that they are likely to do the very thing you asked them not to. Instead, a positive instruction might be, 'Take small steps'. This will be easier for them to translate into appropriate action.

Prevent an escalation

Prevention is by far the most effective behaviour management measure. It can take two forms: *primary* prevention takes a wide view of the overall program and uses high-quality provisions to avoid disruptive behaviours that can arise when children's needs are not being met. It is most suitably used to prevent disengagement, to avoid disputes over scarce play equipment, and to allow children to manage routines. Earlier chapters— particularly Chapter 3—have already covered many of these measures so they will not be repeated here.

A second form of prevention—*secondary* prevention—is where, having noticed that children's play has the potential to become disruptive, you change elements of the situation so that problems that are developing do not surface or those that have appeared do not recur. Secondary prevention can take the form of:

- changing the demands;
- mediating children's learning so that they can engage more successfully;
- shadowing a child who is repeatedly disrupting others.

Change the demands

On occasions, it can help to adjust an activity to make considerate behaviour easier for the children to achieve, rather than expecting the children to change how they are acting. It might be that you cease group time or allow troubled children to withdraw temporarily rather than insisting that they regain command of themselves in a situation that might be stressing them.

Mediate children's engagement

When individual children are disrupting others' play, you can sit with them and help them to settle to a productive activity. This is called *mediation* or *scaffolding* and will both further their learning and avoid repeated assaults on surrounding children. Mediation can also allow you to extend children's stereotypical play such as repeated superhero re-enactments—see Chapter 12.

Shadow troubled children

Instead of joining with individual children at their activity, a more restrictive approach is to have highly disruptive children accompany you during your normal routine. This 'shadowing' of children is not meant to be a punishment but instead offers your moral support while they regain emotional control. Once the children appear calm again, they can return to the social context, perhaps with your help to re-engage through the use of mediation, as described above.

Accede to children's requests

A further strategy is to 'listen with your eyes' and read children's disruptive behaviour or verbal protests as signs that they are not getting their needs met. On occasions when it is possible to grant what they want without violating what you require, and when what they are requesting is reasonable, you can actually change your mind and give them what they are asking for. This is not the same thing as spoiling or 'giving in' to children, which involves giving children something that you believe is unreasonable; being flexible is simply taking into account the new information that what they have asked for means so much to them. You might say something like, 'I didn't realise it meant that much to you. I can see you're very upset that I've said 'No'. So I am thinking about changing my mind'. And if the protests have become loudly tearful, you might add, 'But I can't think with all that noise going on, so once you've calmed down, we can talk about it'.

My research showed that such responsiveness to children's needs had many positive effects (Porter 1999b). It:

- solves the problem: the disruption ceases;
- builds your relationship with the children;
- motivates them to cooperate with your needs on some future occasion, as you have been sensitive and responsive to theirs;
- avoids their rebelling against your directives; and
- allows them to accept those times when you cannot grant what they ask for, particularly when you explain why you have to refuse them.

When the children's request is unreasonable or cannot be accommodated, you can explain why you cannot grant it. When they know that you have listened to them and that you usually try to meet their needs, they will accept the occasional rebuff. Most of the negative reactions we see when children's requests are not granted are a secondary response to being controlled, rather than a reaction to being denied. So within a guidance approach to discipline, the occasional denial will seldom provoke resistance.

Educate children about the effects of their behaviour

Educative measures teach children skills for solving a problem that is giving rise to a disruption. Education can comprise:

- **redirection** to an alternative activity, with a rationale for the suggestion;
- **explanation** of the effect of a behaviour on others; and
- **guided assertion**, in which you help children to speak up for themselves.

Education is appropriate when children do not know the information being imparted or forget to be assertive—but is less successful when an explanation is given repeatedly for the same offence or when children are advised to tell another child to stop a behaviour when they have already done so. Using the same unsuccessful method over and over again only allows the thought-less behaviour to persist, attracting a reputation for the offender and needlessly hurting surrounding children.

At that point, it is safe to assume that the offenders know how they should be behaving (given that you have explained this to them repeatedly) but cannot overcome their emotions and act on that information. In that case, they need assistance to regain emotional control, rather than more information. (Ways to help them to get back in command of themselves are outlined in Chapter 9.)

Guiding principle

You cannot reason with people while they are being unreasonable.

Follow up

When children's assertive messages to a peer are not being heeded or when they report that a peer will not desist, it is clear that they need your help to resolve their dispute. This type of assistance is effective when you can support the children to find their own solutions (using the communication skills described in Chapter 7) and, where necessary, give ideas and suggestions.

Your assistance should involve giving information rather than an accusation. An accusatory tone or message—such as 'I shouldn't have to come over here to help you sort this out' or 'You shouldn't fight with your friends'—often excites secondary reactions in children, such as running away or not abiding by a resolution that has been imposed on them (Porter 1999b). The conflict usually persists for far longer than if the solution is worked out collaboratively.

A second form of follow-up comprises nurturing a child who has been hurt during a dispute. I have found that the most successful way to satisfy the injured child without provoking further aggression from the perpetrator is to withdraw the two children to an area where they can have some privacy, and then to speak to the victim. This method is detailed in Chapter 12.

Reciprocal contracts (or 'deals')

It should be obvious that the term 'reciprocal' is redundant when paired with the term 'contract' because, by their very nature, contracts are reciprocal. If I buy your house, I pay you some money and you give me the title deeds to the property. But most behavioural contracts (or deals) with children specify how the children must behave—and what will happen to them if they do not. Instead, a true deal tells children how you need them to act in a given situation, and also specifies what you will do to help them do so. During story time, for instance, you could agree that the child will sit quietly and negotiate that you will help him do so by letting him choose a book, bring in a favourite book from home, or turn the pages, and by engaging him (and the other children) in a conversation about the events of the story,

Table 8.1: Responses to everyday disruptions

Response	Effective applications	Ineffective applications
Inaction	Inaction can be effective when children: • are being normally exhuberant • act in ways that might irritate adults but which nevertheless harm no one • give vent to strong feelings in inoffensive ways • have already corrected a mistake	Inaction is not advisable: • when the behaviour is disrupting others • when children are not engaged (are reticent) • for exclusion
Defusing resistance • helping children to get started • letting children save face	Defusing resistance can be effective when children: • are only passively resisting directives • are not spontaneously recovering from a mistake	Confrontations with children are more likely to be successfully avoided when adults use a guidance approach to discipline. Children might resist or rebel against an attempt to diffuse their resistance if they perceive adults as controlling
Assertiveness	Assertiveness is useful when children's actions are violating the needs of surrounding individuals and the tone of delivery is informational or matter-of-fact	Assertiveness is ineffective if the feedback is delivered in an accusatory tone
Prevention • **primary**: structuring the program to avoid disruptions • **secondary**: adjusting an activity to make it easier for children to participate without disruptions by: • changing the demands • mediating children's engagement • shadowing troubled children	Primary or secondary prevention can be suitable for: • preventing disengagement • preventing disputes over scarce resources • making routines manageable for the children	Prevention is never inappropriate Secondary prevention is only inappropriate if it is delayed for too long and problems surface in the meantime

(Continued)

Table 8.1: *(Continued)*

Acceding to children's requests	This measure is suitable when the requests are reasonable	Giving children what they ask for is unwise if granting the request would unduly inconvenience others
Education • about the effects of a behaviour on others • about how to be assertive	Education is suitable for: • occasional disruptive acts • to teach children to be assertive about the negative effects of a peer's behaviour	Education is unsuitable for: • repeated outbursts, as the miscreants do not lack information but lack self-control • if the children are already being assertive but the miscreant is not desisting
Follow up to help children solve problems	If too hasty, follow up can interfere with children's independent problem solving	Follow up that is too delayed can allow disputes to escalate and children to be victimised unnecessarily
Contracts	Contracts are suitable for persistent difficulties	To be effective, contracts must specify how adults will help the children to achieve expectations

and so on. It can also help to give active children a discrete fidget item that allows them to move slightly, freeing them to listen.

Conclusion

For most children on most days with most behaviours, the measures described here will be effective, particularly when used with discernment about which approach to employ for which infractions (see Table 8.1). However, when the same children are engaging in the same disruptive pattern over and over again, they almost certainly have been told that this is unacceptable and yet cannot adjust their behaviour to suit the needs of others. This suggests that they lack self-control rather than information about how to act thoughtfully, in which case the suggestions given in Chapter 9 will need to be employed.

9

●●●

Teaching children emotional self-control

Child guidance is a process, the process of assisting children to understand and use constructive behaviors.

GARTRELL (1987: 55)

I believe that growing up is a process of learning that, while we are allowed to feel the full range of emotions, we must express our feelings in ways that do not make us more distressed and do not bother other people. When children cannot act on their feelings without disturbing others, they could be said to be having a *tantrum* (as described in Chapter 6). For the time being, their feelings are out of their control. This chapter contains some ideas for helping them learn—both at the time and in the long term—how to manage their feelings so that they can behave considerately.

Methods to teach self-control

Having so far in this book pointed out the disadvantages of controlling methods of discipline and emphasised the importance of cementing your relationship with children, this chapter describes some nonpunitive means of responding to inconsiderate behaviour, particularly when children have lost control of their emotions.

Explain growing up

Growing up is a process of learning how to be boss of our feelings. Adults (mostly) have learned that we cannot act on every impulse; in contrast,

94

young children believe that if they feel something, it is okay to act on it. This is part of normal development. However, as they are approaching school age, they need to be beginning the life-long process of learning how to be in charge of what they do.

So, I tell children that while their body—their outside—is getting taller, bigger, stronger, and so on, their insides may have forgotten to grow up. Their feelings boss them around and get them into trouble or get them upset (as the case may be). As they are growing up to be a school person shortly— or will be *this* old at their next birthday—now is the right time to start *thinking* about growing up on the inside as well.

You cannot talk children into growing up, or they would not want to do it. Also, you cannot give them suggestions of how they can achieve it. But it can help to warn them that it will take them a long time to think about, but you are sure that part of them knows how to do it. After all, they have grown up on the outside so successfully that this shows that they know how to do it!

While they are thinking about how to teach their feelings to grow up, you will help them when they get out of control. (See the sections below.)

Teach the link between thoughts and feelings

To teach children to manage their emotions, it can be useful to explain to them that their feelings and subsequently their behaviour are controlled by what they *think*. Other people and outside events do not *make* us feel anything: how we think about events leads to our feelings and behaviour. Our feelings help to make life interesting and signal when we need to change some aspect of our lives, but extreme emotions can get in the way of a happy life.

Bill Glasser (1998) says that behaviour has four parts: thinking, feeling, action, and a physiological response (a change in bodily state). It might help to think of these as the four wheels of a front-wheel-drive car. The front two—the driving wheels—are our *thinking* and our *actions*. They pull along behind them our *feelings* and our physical *wellbeing*.

When we wish to go somewhere, we cannot wait until the rear wheels of a car 'get in the mood' to move but instead have to use the front, driving wheels to pull the rear ones along. Likewise, if we want to feel better, we have to change what we think and do—and our feelings and even physical health will improve in turn.

So when children habitually express feelings in ways that interfere with others or with their own social or emotional wellbeing, you can teach them that this comes about because they are thinking is ways that lead to extreme emotions. Some of the common dysfunctional thinking habits are listed in Table 9.1. Once children are aware of the patterns they often use, you can coach them to think in new, more productive ways that, in turn, will lead to more balanced emotional responses.

Table 9.1: Characteristic dysfunctional thinking of children

Thinking style	Common theme	Self-statements	Emotion
Robot thinking	It's not my fault	I can't help it	Feelings of failure
I'm awful	It's all my fault	I can't do anything right because I'm no good	Avoidance of risks
You're awful	It's all your fault	I'd be able to do this if you weren't so horrible	Belligerence
Fairy tale thinking	It's not fair	I wish things would get better (but has no intention of changing own behaviour to bring about improvement)	Hurt Anger
Wimpy thinking (Namby pamby)	I can't stand it	I can't cope if things do not go my way	Anxiety Shyness Over-reaction to threats
Doomsday thinking	It's never going to get better	This always happens Things never work out	Depression

SOURCE: ADAPTED FROM ROUSH (1984, IN KAPLAN & CARTER 1995: 396)

In my conversations with children, I have found that wimpy and doomsday thinking patterns are common to those whose emotions get out of control. Both of these thoughts are often accompanied by one of the other four types—so you will need to explain more than one pattern to troubled children. Wimpy thinking is clearly inaccurate as individuals can 'stand' all sorts of things—even very negative events—and still survive, sometimes happily. And doomsday thinking is inaccurate because *nothing* ever happens always and so things can improve—particularly when children learn to recognise the part they play in their own problems and can change how they are acting.

This method, however, cannot be used at the time when children are upset, as encapsulated in the following guiding principle. Instead, during crises, you will need to use one of the remaining approaches to help children to calm down.

Guiding principle

When a person is drowning that is *not* the time to give swimming lessons.

Faber et al. (1995)

Bring children in close

When babies become upset, we naturally bring them in close to us and soothe them. But often our first impulse with older children is to send them away to sort themselves out alone. That, to my mind, is unfair and is too big a task for young children. (It is even too big a task for many adults.)

So, when children have shown you by their behaviour that they are out of command of their emotions (displaying one of the tantrum types described in Chapter 6), instead of sending them away from you, bring them in close, either physically or psychologically. Cuddle them; soothe them; tell them you understand how badly they are feeling; let them cry—for as long as it takes for them to feel better. Meanwhile, on the grounds that you cannot reason with people while they are being unreasonable, say very little: do not try to hurry them into feeling better nor explain yourself or the problem. That can come later, if at all.

Staying with children tells them that you are willing to help them, even when their behaviour is antisocial. However, sometimes they are too angry to want a cuddle or even your company. In that case, you can still use reflection of feelings (see Chapter 7) to communicate that you understand that they are feeling badly, without bringing them in close physically. You might offer to stay nearby, at a location where you can continue to offer comfort while still supervising the other children, or you might withdraw altogether with the promise that you will return shortly.

For those steeped in a controlling system of discipline, this approach *feels* like a reward for poor behaviour. However, the goal under a guidance approach is merely to teach children a necessary skill—namely, how to get back in control of their emotions. Remaining close to them does not do that task for them, but it does give them the support they need to achieve it. This provides a safety net for those times when they feel out of control of themselves.

Sometimes, when you bring children in close to you, their feelings escalate into a protesting tantrum (see Chapter 6). If you are able to cuddle them in a nurturing manner throughout this, they might go through a series of emotions before resolving their feelings. Typically, they alternate between anger, sadness, and bargaining with you (that is, reporting that they are alright now, when they clearly are not yet) until, finally, they will become truly calm (Robinson, pers. comm.). However, if they do not want your physical support as they experience these emotions or if they are thrashing about wildly and could injure you, you must withdraw and return to them when they have calmed down on their own.

This protesting tantrum is less common than you might think, however. If your talk to that point has been non-accusatory, has sympathised with how upset the children are feeling and asked their advice about how you can help, it is less likely that you will provoke the protesting tantrum as it is, after all, only a secondary reaction to being dominated.

Provide time away

Sometimes, you cannot or do not want to accompany children while they calm down, in which case time out might seem an attractive option. This usually involves isolating a child on a chair that is somewhat separate from others and asking him or her to think about a transgression. The child is typically allowed to leave when able to state what he or she did 'wrong' or should have done instead, or when adults judge that the child has calmed down sufficiently; less commonly, a predetermined time limit is imposed. However, time out in these forms has many disadvantages:

- it isolates hysterical children;
- they might damage the area where they have been isolated;
- they can create a lot of noise that does not give you the break you need;
- they might forget that they are being punished;
- you might forget about the children and leave them in isolation for too long;
- it causes them to resent adults who impose this form on punishment on them; and
- when you are separated from children, you cannot give them the emotional support they need to calm down.

As a result, time out will not work to discourage inconsiderate behaviour. However, you can use time away instead to give both yourself and the child some time to regain your composure.

To help understand this alternative, picture a situation where you have become distressed. I assume that, in order to feel better you might talk the problem over with a friend, go for a walk, listen to music, turn on the TV, have a sleep, or perhaps read a good book. Whatever method you choose, it is a safe bet that you *do not* place yourself on a chair in the bathroom facing a wall in the hopes that this will improve your mood!

So it is with children. When they have become distressed, they need to do something pleasant and have some solitude to help them regain their emotional balance. Therefore when children's behaviour tells you that they cannot cope, you can suggest that they go off by themselves until they feel better. They might enjoy putting on some favourite music in a quiet corner of the room, selecting a book to read, resting on some cushions, or looking out the window.

This is not a punishment: children should find their solitude enjoyable and refreshing. If they perceive it as a punishment—like time out—it will not work and may even provoke secondary reactions such as destroying the area where they are placed. (If these secondary reactions occur, either you are using a controlling style and do not realise it, or the children are so accustomed to being controlled that they are reacting negatively even though you are using guidance methods. In this case, it can help to reflect their feelings (see Chapter 7), reassure them that you want to help them to feel better, and ask how they would like you to help.)

To those steeped in a tradition of rewards and punishment, this pleasant time away experience can seem as if you are giving children a reward for thoughtless behaviour. You might think that other children will act thoughtlessly just so they too can have some time away. However, as being distressed is distressing, no one would voluntarily choose to feel that way just to earn some solitude, especially when they have access to personal space in the normal course of events. Furthermore, it is not an issue of punishing children for becoming distressed: that is a natural childhood event and so, as I have said before, to punish them for feeling overwhelmed would be to punish them for being children. All you need to do is teach them that they can overcome their feelings in positive ways, without being terrified by them. Behavioural mistakes are an opportunity for teaching, not for punishment.

Warn about relapses

Occasionally, children's behaviour improves and then they take a step backwards again. Expect this. You can use relapses as a reminder that the children know how to control their feelings: they did it once and can do it again. Relapses can thus be regarded as a type of test to see if you both can get yourselves back on track again to overcome the problem.

Guidelines for teaching self-control

Step in early. Often a passive tantrum (whingeing/whining or unco-operativeness) comes before an active (protesting or social) tantrum. So it will be quicker and more humane if you can comfort children during passive tantrums before these build up into the more active forms.

Use minimal talk. When children are out of control of their feelings, their behaviour is a sign that they are already too stressed to listen to us. At times like this, it will only make matters worse if you try to reason with them. Wait until they are calm, and talk then. Usually, though, you do not have to explain later, because the children knew all along—they just couldn't act on the information—and now that they have overcome their feelings, they do not need you to preach at them.

Children will give off non-verbal signs when you are talking too much. They might roll their eyes up, or get 'That Look' which makes you want to demand in exasperation: 'And you can get that look off your face as well!'. Another is what Steve Biddulph (1993) calls the Mona Lisa smile; finally, some youngsters smirk or give off a 'Go your hardest' type of swagger. When they do this, stop talking: start acting.

Give repeated opportunities for practice. Give out-of-control children as many opportunities as possible to practise getting back in command of themselves. On the other hand, when you really *cannot* give them help, you do not have to and can say so: 'I can see you're feeling upset, and I wish I could help you to calm down, but I can't just now. I am sorry'.

I find an analogy useful here: if you give children swimming lessons every day for two weeks, they might learn to swim in that time; if you give them lessons once a month, they might take a year to become competent swimmers. This tells us that the more practice children can get at learning a new skill, the more quickly they will learn it—but either way, they still do achieve it. So if you cannot give children help to calm down every time they need it, there will be other opportunities to do so: nothing is surer than that they will lose the plot again and will be able to practise controlling their feelings then. Consistency is unnecessary, therefore; but repeated practice helps.

Accept their feelings, but not their actions. You must be clear with children that it is quite okay for them to feel angry: do not tell them to calm down and be quiet. The issue is not that they are angry but that they have been acting on those feelings in inconsiderate ways.

Keep them comfortable. It will be hard for children who are tantruming to calm down when they are uncomfortably hot. Offer to place a cool facecloth on their temples or help them to strip off their outer clothing if they want you to, so that physical discomfort does not add to their distress.

Encourage them. Reassure them that you believe they can do it—they *can* calm down. When I have talked with the children beforehand about growing up, I've mentioned all the things that they have already learned to do, and told them that I have faith that they can learn to manage their feelings as well. Then, while I am supporting them to settle, I say things like, 'Take your time. I know you'll be able to calm down when you're ready. I *know* you can do it. I believe in you'.

Go the distance. Unless interrupted, be certain to last out until the children are truly calm so that they have had enough time to get back in command of their feelings. Otherwise, they will get into more trouble straight away.

Do not punish. If you attempt to force children to regain their composure, be warned: it does not work. Your response must be nurturing, so that the children learn that emotions are not terrifying, that they do have the skills to overcome their distress and that they will receive support if they temporarily lose control of themselves.

Get medical advice. You cannot expect children to take emotional charge of behaviour that has a medical cause, so unwell children will need medical interventions. Also, you will need medical advice about the safety of allowing children to get out of control of their emotions if they have illnesses such as a heart condition or asthma that are aggravated by emotional stress.

Conclusion

Some children do not want to grow up because they believe that adults have no fun. They might perceive all the adults in their life as stressed and permanently tired, so it can help to talk with children about what you enjoy about being older—such as having more independence than you did as a child, and enjoying adult toys such as the gadgets and your car—and also to be playful in your interactions with them so that they see you enjoying life. This gives them some incentive to grow up and take increasing responsibility for themselves, without which they will resist learning how to take command of their feelings.

10

• •

Resolving chronic difficulties

You cannot solve the problem with the same kind of thinking that has created the problem.

ALBERT EINSTEIN (IN DE SHAZER 1993: 84)

It is obvious that problems persist because the attempts to solve them have not worked. This is not to say that the attempts were misguided: they might have worked with another child, a different behaviour, or at some other time. But, for some reason, they are not working now.

If you have been dealing with children's inconsiderate behaviour in a way that you expect would have worked—and it has not—the following recommendations might give you some additional ideas.

Check your preventive measures

When a disruptive behaviour is persisting, it can help to check that the program is mostly meeting the children's needs (see Chapter 3). It is also worth considering whether the behaviour could be communicating a need. Individual children might have atypical development that puts them out of step with their playmates; they might be stressed, being abused, feeling unwell, or taking responsibility for adult issues (such as a parent's emotional wellbeing) that are stretching their coping skills; or they might have language or other delays that make it difficult for them to self-instruct and thus govern their own behaviour. Once you can identify what is troubling children, you might be able to target an intervention more accurately.

Fine-tune your interventions

Given that behavioural difficulties have persisted even after accurate and skilful intervention, it is likely that, unwittingly, the intervention—which was intended to solve the problem obviously—actually *is* the problem. The purest example of this is when behaviours are secondary reactions to a controlling style of discipline that has been in place. This can be reversed by instigating a guidance approach.

The second possibility is that adults have conscientiously, consistently, and diligently been applying the same solution over and over again. In that case, a change in solution is called for. This is not to say that a whole new intervention will need to be planned because, like the snowball growing in size as it rolls down the hill, a small but crucial change in an intervention can be enough to change from a vicious to a virtuous cycle of behaviour-and-correction. In the vein of singer Paul Kelly's observation that 'From little things, big things grow' the remaining interventions aim to fine-tune—rather than overturn—previous interventions.

Start with an easier behaviour

When children display many disruptive behaviours, common sense might suggest intervening with the one that is most troublesome. But I suggest you start with an easier behaviour, get some success with that, and then deal with the next—if it is still a problem. Sometimes, while you are dealing with the first behaviour, the children learn what you expect and develop a warmer relationship in which they *want* to please you, and the other problems go away. But if not and you have to attend to the original issue after all, at least you and the children have already developed some confidence about your successes so far. An example is beginning to deal with uncooperative behaviour during playtime, rather than at sleep time when children's protests would interrupt those who are sleeping.

Reframe your understanding of the problem

Your response to children's behaviour will depend on what you think the behaviour *means*. But if your approach is not working, maybe your explanation of the behaviour is not helping. The most common explanations that do not help are those that blame children's personalities for the behaviour or blame the behaviour on something that has happened in the past. Because personalities and the past cannot be changed, these types of explanations cause you to lose hope that things can improve.

> **Guiding principle**
> Focus on present conditions that maintain the problem, not past causes (as the past cannot be changed).

So, to find a new solution, you will need to find a new way of looking at the problem. A new view of the problem is called a *reframe*. Reframing is performed in the following steps:

1. **Describe what is occurring.** Note what the children do and when they do it.
2. **Describe present corrective attempts.** Describe who gets involved in trying to correct the behaviour and what their responses entail. Identify the usual effects of these measures.
3. **Identify the explanation that has led to previous corrective attempts.** Explanations that do not work usually comprise one of two ideas: first, that the children are 'doing it deliberately' (perhaps even 'to get at you'), which will have led to a range of responses all designed to make them stop it. The second explanation is that the children cannot help themselves (because of their personality, disability, or events in the past). This idea will have led to walking around them like you are walking on eggshells, avoiding making demands on them. This is usually alternated with exasperation, but that too has little effect.
4. **Generate a new explanation.** A new view of the problem will look at what is maintaining the behaviour *now*, rather than what might have triggered it originally. For instance, when children appear to be socially immature in that they cannot separate from their parents, it could be that they are trying to look after a distressed parent and therefore cannot be apart. This view regards them as exercising too much responsibility, rather than too little autonomy. Or, children might be unclear that you will insist on thoughtful behaviour when you are busy, so instead of regarding their behaviour as 'attention-seeking' and ignoring it, you can regard it as an attempt to clarify expectations, which you can do by becoming focused on the behaviour and its correction.
5. **Change how you respond.** The new view of the problem will enable you to let go of an ineffective solution so that you can try another instead (Fisch et al. 1982).

When you are reframing, keep in mind that you cannot diagnose the intent behind children's behaviour as you cannot read minds: you are simply looking at the *effect* of their behaviour. Realising that behaviour would cease if it were ineffective, you can assume that it is being maintained because it works in some way. For instance, children who disrupt group story time might be the 'group barometer'—that is, the one who signals when everyone has had enough.

A simple example of reframing is when children are accustomed to intimidating or manipulating adults. If this has been happening, it can help to tell them firmly, 'You don't scare me'. A clear gaze and a calm voice while delivering this surprising message can be a very powerful way to let the children know that you will not be dissuaded from requiring considerate behaviour.

Interrupt the pattern

Let's say that you cannot figure out a new view or reframe of a recurring problem. In that case, you could simply use another approach called 'pattern interruption' (Durrant 1995). With this approach, you allow the behaviour to continue, on the understanding that it is helping the children in some way, even if you do not understand how. In line with the principles of guidance, you cannot frustrate children's legitimate needs—but you can insist that the resulting behaviour is less disruptive to others (Molnar & Lindquist 1989).

There is an old saying that a chain is only as strong as its weakest link. With this in mind, you can break up the chain or sequence of events that occurs whenever the children's behaviour is disruptive, producing in its place a new pattern. To disrupt the old, dysfunctioning pattern you could (Durrant 1995):

- change the location of the behaviour;
- change who is involved;
- change the sequence of the steps involved;
- add a new element;
- introduce random starting and stopping;
- increase the frequency of the behaviour.

So, when children throw themselves down on the floor in a tantrum, as long as you can do so safely, you could move them to some cushions so that they are more comfortable (changing the location); you could invite children who often fight over their toys in the sandpit, to argue now before they go outside so that they do not miss out once outdoor play time begins (changing the sequence or introducing random starting); you could let children know that it's okay to cry when their parent leaves and that they can continue to do so for as long as it takes for them to feel better (increasing the frequency of the crying), and so on.

Even when you do not understand why the children persist with their behaviours, changing the sequence of events will alter the behaviour into a form that is less disruptive.

Try a reversal

If all else has failed, try doing the opposite of what you have been doing so far (Amatea 1989), even if you do not understand in advance how that could help. If you have been ignoring the behaviour, give it your attention. If you have been sending children away to sort themselves out, bring them in close to you and give them your support to get back in control of themselves. If you have been trying to talk them out of a behaviour, give them permission to continue with it—as long as it does not bother anyone. If you have been thinking that they cannot help themselves, notice the times when the behaviour does not occur, and expect them to do more of what causes those exceptions.

This suggestion to do something different is based on the advice: 'Always change a losing game' (Fisch et al. 1982: 88). Or, put another way:

Guiding principle

If something isn't working, don't do it again.

DE SHAZER ET AL. (1986: 212)

Look for exceptions

When a problem has been occurring for a long time, it is easy to believe that it is 'always' happening. But nothing ever happens 100% of the time: there will inevitably be times when the children do not display the troublesome behaviour, in which case your job is to help them examine what is different about those occasions compared with the times when the behaviour occurs.

The notion of 'positive blame' can be useful here. In remarking on the times when they *have* behaved considerately, you can ask children, 'How did you get that to happen?' (Kral & Kowalski 1989). If they claim that the considerate behaviour was just a fluke, you can ask them whether they think the fluke might happen again (Molnar & de Shazer 1987). This implies that they are in charge of making the exceptions happen.

Another option for children who believe that they are not in control of their own behaviour (the robot thinkers) is to pose the miracle question: 'If you woke up tomorrow and a miracle had happened overnight and this problem was fixed, what would be different?' You can use this for older children who wet the bed, for instance. Once they can describe what they would be doing if the problem were fixed, you can invite them to have a go at doing that behaviour and see if it helps.

Give up strategically

Particularly when you feel that you have tried 'everything' to solve a chronic problem, it can be useful to give up: to abandon all efforts and place responsibility for solving the problem back on the child. This is because trying 'everything' usually entails 'everything we can think of to make the child stop it'. But the more you try to *make* children stop acting in a particular way, the more responsible *you* become for their actions, and the less responsible *they* have to be. So, in these circumstances, tell children that you are giving up: you have run out of ideas. If they have any suggestions, you are willing to listen but in the meantime, when they act thoughtlessly, you will do whatever it takes (within reason) to get through the crisis. If the children do not like your solution, you can invite them to come up with a better idea about how to solve their behaviour.

Have fun

By the time children's behaviour has become a serious problem, life has got very earnest. Caregivers begin feeling frustrated—even desperate—and, because you are human, you might dislike the children who cause you to feel that way. Meanwhile, they feel victimised by being told off all the time. One thing is for sure: no one is having any fun. So, if nothing else has worked, at least you can have some fun: when a child is throwing a tantrum, you could perform an ethnic dance, have a tantrum yourself, sing at the top of your lungs, or do a handstand—whatever. There isn't a child worth his or her salt who can carry on with a tantrum while you're making a fool of yourself. And if it doesn't fix the behaviour, at least you've enjoyed yourself.

Conclusion

When something is not working, it is very foolish to do more of it in the hopes that this will improve matters. If your present solutions were going to work, they would have by now. So dismiss notions from the controlling approaches that you should do something unsuccessful more consistently— and instead try a new approach, even if at first you do not know how that could help. If that does not produce an improvement, secure the parents' permission to consult a specialist in children's behaviour so that persistent difficulties do not disadvantage miscreants and the surrounding adults and children.

Suggested further reading

Although no texts are written for early childhood on the category of interventions recommended in this chapter, a useful school-based text is:

Durrant, M. (1995). *Creative strategies for school problems.* Epping, NSW: Eastwood Family Therapy Centre/New York: Norton.

Part Four

●●●

Specific behavioural challenges of young children

Any approach to discipline is judged to be a failure not only on the obvious criterion that it fails to establish and affect appropriate standards of behaviour, but also if, in establishing such standards, it does so primarily by teaching children to obey rules rather than to make reasoned judgments about what actions are desirable, and about how actually to decide to act in those desirable ways.

COVALESKIE (1992: 175)

Part Four applies the guidelines and general recommendations given in earlier chapters to some behavioural challenges that are common in the early childhood years. Many of the behaviours are understandable, given the children's developmental stage. But when the behaviours are happening too often, at the wrong time or place, or are still present at a later age than usual, you will need to take some action to help the children to progress beyond them.

Which responses you choose to employ will depend on what you have already tried. If a behaviour has been difficult for some time, it might be useful to use the opposite strategy to what you have been trying so far. On the other hand, sometimes a slight change in flavour—what I call 'fine-tuning' a method that you are already using—can be enough of a difference to make a difference, without having to instigate a completely new management plan.

If the ideas given here do not help, do not persist with the same approach. If a problem—even a small one—goes on for too long, it can become the whole focus of the centre, and children who are experiencing the problem can quickly develop a reputation among peers that interferes with their social inclusion. If you have run out of ideas, ask the children's parents for permission to consult a specialist in children's behaviour so that you can nip the problem in the bud before it becomes a habit.

Many of the behavioural challenges discussed in the coming chapters are typical for young children. This means that the children do not need 'fixing' as they are not broken (Gowen & Nebrig 2002): they simply need to be responded to thoughtfully and with sensitivity so that they learn from the guidance they receive.

11

· ·

Disruptions during routines

When we think clearly about what we want for children, our own and other people's, it is obvious that we want them to grow up to be our peers. If we could keep that fact in the forefront of our attitudes towards children, we might avoid many of the fruitless battles and instead serve as guides, welcomers, and protectors as children make their valiant efforts to grow up and join us.

WARREN (1977, IN STONEHOUSE 1988: 13)

The task of managing self-care activities with increasing independence is quite demanding on children and their adult supervisors. But although it could be tempting to set up invariant routines to make these more orderly, a key function of meal times and other routine activities is educational and so they must provide opportunities for children to make choices and exercise autonomy.

When a task is difficult, it can help to simplify the process so that success is more probable. As performing tasks in large groups can be challenging to young children, it can also help to ensure that all staff are on duty and to minimise the number of children who are being required to perform the routine simultaneously, so that it is more manageable for them.

Meal times

In terms of behavioural disruptions, hungry young children are less likely to cope with the demands of their day. Therefore, their meals need to give them enough fuel. However, food is more than fuel for children's physical, social, emotional and cognitive development: it is also a human rights issue in that children deserve food that meets their nutritional and cultural requirements and satisfies their preferences.

Birch et al. (1999: 199–200) report that 'The emotional tone of the social interactions surrounding feeding can shape children's food-acceptance patterns'. Thus, to encourage sound eating habits and to facilitate interactions among children and between caregivers and children, meal times have to be pleasant and comfortable.

Enjoyment. Eating is an important source of enjoyment for most adults; children should similarly find meals pleasant (NCAC 1993). Therefore, you must avoid allowing your concern for children's nutrition or use of manners to intrude on the pleasure of meal times (NCAC 1993).

Choice. The second criterion for high-quality meal times is that the children be given choice about their food. The highest level of choice is allowing children to determine when they feel hungry and thus want to eat. This can be done by serving meals on just a couple of tables and allowing individual children to partake when they feel hungry, then replenishing with new servings for the next round. This might not be manageable for all hot meals but could be possible for snacks.

The second level of choice is allowing children to select how much and what type of food to eat (obviously from a restricted range). This can be done by placing a bowl in the centre of each table and allowing the children to serve their own portions themselves. This gives them autonomy, allowing them to choose how much to eat and how many serves to take (within reason).

Interaction. The third criterion for a high-quality meal time is that it permits interaction among the children and between the children and staff. Seating arrangements can foster conversations among the children. In line with the advice to offer choice where possible, children could be permitted to choose where to sit. However, this can raise three problems: first, the children can spend a good deal of time in dispute over who will sit next to whom; second, there can be a lot of milling about as individual children try to locate a place to sit; third, particular pairs or groupings of children can disrupt each other throughout the meal so might be better to be separated. You might therefore choose, say, to determine where children will sit for meal times, perhaps clustering friends together or asking the children with whom they would like to sit, while allowing the children to decide where to sit for the shorter snack times. Alternatively, you might designate the table at which children sit, while the children can independently choose their precise seat placement.

To foster communication between caregivers and children, caregivers should sit with the children at meal times. This provides some supervision and, more importantly, allows adults and children to chat about topics of interest to the children. This relationship building is, of course, valuable in its own right but is also useful for discipline in that the children are more willing to please an adult whom they know and who takes an interest in them.

Meanwhile, the caregivers should eat with the children. Perhaps in an attempt to save on food costs, some centres do not allow staff to eat the food that has been prepared for the children. However, allowing them to do so avoids having hungry adults try to rush children through their meal so that the adults can get their own lunch. And when the adults eat the same meal as the children, this communicates to the children that the food is enjoyable. (If the adults do not like it, this should signal a change of menu.)

Fussy eating

Even when the meals you provide are culturally and individually appropriate for the children, there will be times when individual children refuse to eat what has been prepared for them. Throughout the development of the human race, being suspicious of new foods has ensured our survival (Birch et al. 1995). For example, it is possible that children's preference for sweet food might be part of our species' make-up as, in the wild, sweet things are seldom poisonous (Birch et al. 1999). This means that it is natural that young children will be fussy eaters until they become familiar with a range of foods and realise that these are safe.

Ask the children to taste—not necessarily to eat. You might ask the children to taste the set meal in order to educate their taste buds. But forcing them to eat it can make them resistant to that food even if otherwise they might have liked it.

Provide a substitute (within reason). It pays to have something else as a stand-by for the children to eat instead. Some caregivers object to offering children alternative food on the grounds that it will only encourage them to be fussy eaters if they know they can have something else. However, it is not acceptable to allow children to go hungry.

Adjust the menu. If refusals are common to many children, a change in the menu is indicated, not least to satisfy the children but also because wasted food is expensive. If just one or two children are refusing to eat the meals, you could consult their parents for their suggestions. Children who are especially fussy eaters can still be encouraged to eat the centre's meals but perhaps the parents themselves could provide a snack as back-up in case their child refuses to eat.

Be alert for food intolerances. Another reason not to force children to eat the prepared food is that sometimes they refuse food because it upsets their body. They cannot tell you this, but somehow they know to avoid particular foods. This can result in refusing a certain class of foods. More likely, however, is that children with intolerances will simply notice that food in general upsets them and so they become anxious about all foods (although keep in mind that being somewhat suspicious of foods is natural in young children). These children are likely to be small for their age.

The opposite pattern comes about because food to which we are intolerant gives us a quick 'fix' or pick-up, followed by a let-down. To avoid the withdrawal effect, the children need another dose of the same food. The pattern, then, is that they will choose the same food or food category over and over, will ask for particular foods when tired as these will pick them up, and might be constantly eating, resulting in becoming overweight.

Three categories of foods are the most suspect: children with a family history of allergies (such as asthma, eczema or migraines) can be sensitive to whole foods—that is, dairy products, eggs, wheat, corn, cereals and caffeine (in chocolate, coke, tea and coffee). The second class of triggers for food sensitivities are additives such as colourings and preservatives; and the third class are naturally-occurring chemicals and foods such as sugars, salicylates, MSG (chemical number 621) and amines.

If you notice either of these patterns of fussy eating in individual children, it might help to talk with their parents to see if they want to investigate possible food sensitivities. If found, it will be necessary to accommodate the children's particular dietary requirements as this will avoid medical complications and also erratic behaviour arising from a reaction to particular foods.

Another possibility is that the children are copying their parents' attitude to food. If a parent is constantly on a diet or has anorexia, for instance, the child might learn that food is dangerous and so will avoid eating. Again, this is a subject that you could raise tactfully with parents if you think this might apply to a child in your care.

Discuss inside growing up. Some children who are fussy eaters have simply never exposed themselves to different foods often enough to learn to like them. For these children, you might introduce the idea that, although their outside has grown up to be the age they are in years (let's say, four-years-old), their tummy has forgotten to grow up so that it can eat four-year-old foods. See Chapter 9 for more detail on this approach.

Do not use rewards. Meal time can be a valuable time for teaching children how to notice when they are hungry and when they have eaten enough so that they become internally cued when it comes to food, rather than eating in response to external cues even when they are not hungry. So you must avoid using external controls to shape children's eating, as focusing on external consequences will undermine children's ability to regulate their food intake according to their body's (internal) needs. Therefore you should not reward children for eating and neither should you chastise them for not eating. You might ask them, 'Is your body not hungry right now, or just not hungry for pasta?'. If the children say that they are not hungry, perhaps you could set aside a bowl of food for them to eat later; if they are not hungry for this particular meal, you will need to offer a substitute.

It has been a common practice to use children's favourite food (such as dessert) as a reward for eating foods that they dislike. This is unwise, as food rewards have the opposite effect to what we aim for—namely, they make the undesired food appear *less* attractive than it already seemed (Birch et al. 1999).

Obtain nutritional or medical advice. When children are underweight or sickly, this can add extra pressure on you to help them to eat. Sometimes, your concerns for their health will be justified while at other times, their eating pattern is not compromising their health and so you are concerning yourself unnecessarily. To avoid this, you might ask their parents to consult a doctor for an overall health check for their child. If the children are recommended to have a vitamin or mineral supplement, this will assuage some of your concerns about their health and relieve you of the obligation to pressure them to eat as the supplements will fulfil their nutritional requirements while they are learning to eat a wider range of foods.

Sleep times

Managing sleep times is always going to be a challenge. If you do not ensure that tired children have a sleep, they are likely to be disruptive later out of sheer exhaustion. If, however, you force them to sleep, you are in for a prolonged period of issuing commands that might destroy your rapport with the children and thus undermine your subsequent disciplinary efforts.

Maintain home routines. It will help if you can use similar forms of assistance (such as patting or low music) as parents use at home and allow children to bring in a favourite soft toy, pillow or pacifier from home. Once they are beginning no longer to need afternoon naps, you will need to decide in collaboration with parents when to stop insisting on these. But even during this transition phase, it will be important to allow children to sleep if they report being tired; otherwise, they might be out of sorts for the remainder of the day.

Minimise numbers. An effective way to ensure that you are not trying to get all the children to go to sleep simultaneously is to schedule sleep time immediately after lunch. As the children will finish eating at differing times, you can give each one support individually when they first come to lie down.

Make rest time a comfort zone. It can help to place the children in the same location each day so that they develop a sense of comfort with the area where they are being asked to rest.

Do not force children to sleep. You can require children to have a rest but have no power to force them to sleep. So if individual children seem unable to go to sleep with the usual assistance, you might have to give permission for them simply to rest, maybe while looking at some books.

Use disciplinary measures at other times. Sometimes, children's refusal to sleep is part of an overall pattern of uncooperative behaviour. However, it is difficult to deal with while other children are trying to get to sleep as the ensuing noise will disturb them. It can pay, therefore, to deal with the uncooperative behaviour at more convenient times, thus teaching the children that they are to take your directives seriously and teaching them to overcome their distaste for certain tasks. Then, at sleep time, there will be fewer disruptions, without your having to intervene specifically at that time.

Provide for the non-sleepers. If there are children who do not need a sleep, they must be separated from those who are sleeping to avoid interfering with others' getting to sleep and so that non-sleepers do not have to be too restrained in their play. Meanwhile, non-sleepers continue to need active supervision and mediation of their play, as otherwise they might wander around aimlessly and not engage in a productive way with the activities.

Group time disruptions

Group time tends to attract two sorts of difficulties: children who prefer not to participate and so disrupt others by touching or escaping the session; and those who are so enticed by the activity that they rise up on their knees, thus blocking the view of the child behind them. In my observations, disruptions from disengaged children are the more common difficulty, becoming more likely the longer sessions continue (Porter 1999b).

Reading aloud to children is intended to teach them about the act of reading and about how to make sense of story sequences (Conlon 1992). However, my research supported Katz's (1995) observation that early childhood educators seriously overestimate children's academic skills and underestimate their intellectual skills. By forcing children to sit still and listen, we are asking them to do something that is academically challenging; when we do this at the age of two or three years, it is far too demanding. The concern is that while we might be imparting particular content (assuming that the content is educational), we might unwittingly be teaching children that language activities are dull. And it is worse to dislike learning than to be ignorant.

My research into behaviour management in child (day) care centres showed that if disengaged children are not attracted by the activities of the group, it only provokes secondary difficulties if caregivers force them to attend. Instead, caregivers should change both the content and process of group time.

Make group time voluntary. The ideal situation would be to make group time voluntary. Voluntary sessions would look like this: a caregiver would ask one or two children if they would like a story. As the children become captivated, others would come up to join the group also. When you read high-quality books and lead challenging songs, most children on most days would choose to participate.

Voluntary participation raises three issues, the first being what to do about the children who never choose to take part. This is usually because there is a mismatch between the language used during the session and the children's comprehension levels: the language is too simple for gifted children, or too advanced for children with language impairments or those for whom English is their second language. One solution might be for you to bring to the sessions a form listing each child's name and to check attendance on this form, thereby monitoring which children seldom attend and thus identifying those who need individual language sessions in some other format, such as one-on-one story reading or remedial language sessions.

A second issue is when caregivers would take their breaks, if not during group sessions. However, group sessions are intended for educational purposes so the timetabling issues have to be overcome by other means.

The third objection that is often raised is, 'How do we get children ready to sit in groups at school if we do not force them to do so in their early childhood years?'. My response is that we want young people to learn to drive a car when they are 16, but we do not expect them to learn it during early childhood. So it is for academic skills. Children will achieve these when the time is right. And if they do not, they might not be quite ready for school; or school is demanding too much for the children's age—in which case, schools would need to change their own practices rather than dictating developmentally inappropriate practices to the early childhood sector.

Supply fidget items. Children with sensory integration difficulties will not be able to sit still *and* listen (Soden, pers. comm.). These children need to be allowed to fidget discretely with squishy toys. This small amount of movement will keep their nervous systems calm enough to be able to listen. (See Soden 2002a, 2002b.)

Minimise waiting time. As well as being attractive to the children, group time must be highly organised; otherwise, it occasions a good deal of waiting. As few children are able to sit and do nothing, waiting time becomes a major motivational and behavioural issue.

Minimise the duration. If group times are too long, the children become focused on the desire to escape and on the caregiver's domination of them (Alger 1984). A good rule to work by is that children's concentration span for adult-initiated activities is likely to be three minutes multiplied by their age in years. Thus, the duration of group sessions for three-year-olds should not exceed nine minutes; and 12 minutes for four-year-olds. Not only will this duration maximise the children's participation during the session but it will also facilitate an orderly transition to the next activity (Alger 1984).

Restrict group size. Reading aloud with children is also intended to satisfy their emotional needs for closeness and conversation (Conlon 1992). This is impossible to do in large groups. Field and Boesser (2002) recommend that children be involved in groups that number one more than they have had birthdays: in other words, four children per group of three-year olds; five children for four-year-olds. Although this is clearly impracticable in child care centres, it does give an indication of how demanding it is to expect children to participate in sessions of ten or 15 children. Awareness of this might help you to tolerate their distractability.

Allow children to depart. If you have an obligatory group session, nevertheless, allow restless children to depart—as long as they can do so without disrupting others. When children know that they can leave, those who stay will voluntarily manage their own behaviour. And if one child's departure initiates a general exodus from the group, that will be valuable information about how demanding the session has become. All of us have experienced planning an activity that we were sure would excite the children, only to find that it fell flat. You will have to accept the children's verdict, not yours, so if the children 'vote with their feet' by leaving, you can use that information to help plan your program in the future.

Toileting

It is uncommon for children to be toilet trained successfully before the age of two years and three months and, even at this age, they are really toilet timed, responding to frequent reminders from adults to go to the toilet (or bathroom), rather than deciding for themselves that they need to go.

Minimise pressure on training. Sometimes, when adults become anxious about toilet training or want their child to be trained by a certain date, the children pick up on their anxiety and in turn refuse to be trained at all. So it is important to avoid toilet learning becoming a major focus of your program (Greenman & Stonehouse 1997). If you feel that individual children are under a little too much pressure to learn toileting, perhaps you could tactfully suggest to the parents that everyone backs off for a few weeks, and start again later.

Explain inside growing up. In the meantime you could explain to children that they are growing up on the outside, which tells you that they will soon ready to grow up on the inside as well, by learning to do a wee like a big three-year-old (or whatever age they will be at their next birthday).

Expect setbacks. Some children acquire toileting skills quite successfully until they turn three and then they have a series of accidents again. This comes about because, now that they are three, they can concentrate for a longer time on what they are doing and so there are not as many natural interruptions during which they could notice that they need to go to the toilet. You might deal with this by reminding children that needing to do a wee can sneak up on them and so they will need to think extra hard to remember to be boss of their sneaky wee's. You can also revert to the earlier toilet-timing method of suggesting that they go to the toilet at natural breaks, until they regain control of their toileting for themselves.

Do not use rewards or punishments. It is important not to punish children for toileting accidents. On the other hand, do not praise or reward successes either (say, with a sweet or stars on a chart). If we tell children that they are 'good' girls or boys when they use the potty or toilet, this implies that they are 'bad' when they have an accident. Furthermore, reward systems such as star charts make you more responsible for their behaviour than they are and, as with all rewards, children can come to resent being manipulated. Rewards also take the focus away from the fact that the children are learning some new competencies, shifting attention instead to the receipt of the reward. Therefore, acknowledge children's achievements, giving informative but not evaluative feedback (see Chapter 4).

Separating from parents

Children will differ in how often and how young they were when they first separated from their parents. They will also differ in the strategies they have developed to cope and in the circumstances in which they have been placed previously (Waters 1996). This means that children will react differently to separating from their parents when they begin child care or preschool.

Some youngsters will enjoy the early days in the centre but then, when they realise that the arrangement is permanent, they develop problems; other children have separation problems from the beginning. Sometimes, a new stage of cognitive development signals a new understanding of being left in care and separation difficulties begin unexpectedly after some months (Greenman & Stonehouse 1997).

Preparation. At enrolment, talk with parents about how they would like you to respond to any separation difficulties and how they plan to handle these themselves (Greenman & Stonehouse 1997). Ask how their child has responded to previous separations and what they think will work for their child if separation problems occur, and also pass on your suggestions.

A staggered start, with frequent visits before their actual start date can help, but many parents do not find or do not use child care until the last minute before they return to paid employment, with the result that some children are introduced into care abruptly.

You can ask parents to bring in their child's favourite comforter from home, and try to give the children some favourite activities and foods, especially in the early days. If it can be arranged, beginning with only a small group of other children of their age can also help.

Suggest that the parent joins with the child before she goes. It can help if the parent and child find a quiet corner in which to have a close hug so that they join emotionally before separating. In the busy-ness of getting out of the house, parents are not always able to give their children the emotional closeness they need to get through the day.

Recommend that parents keep goodbyes brief. Suggest that the parent states briefly and calmly that she is leaving now, and hand the child over to a familiar caregiver. Encourage parents to leave once they say they are going, and not to return (Greenman & Stonehouse 1997). If this means that parents have had to leave a distressed child with you, invite them to call you later to check on the child.

A structured goodbye routine can be useful when children often have difficulty accepting the departure of their parent. It might be that the children put their bag in its place, are helped by their parent to begin an activity, have a hug, and then the parent leaves. It might help to make the children active in saying goodbye, perhaps by opening the door for the parent (Greenman & Stonehouse 1997).

Ensure that parents *never* sneak out on children when they are leaving, even if warning the children that they are going leads to an outburst of emotion. If children have no warning signals to distinguish when they have to be self-reliant versus when someone is available to comfort them, they will be anxious all the time. Also, suggest that parents *tell* their child they are leaving: if they *ask* if that's okay, the children are likely to say 'no', leaving everyone frustrated and miserable and the children feeling betrayed as their parent will go anyway.

Allocate a primary caregiver. To help settle new or distressed children, you can allocate one person to be their primary caregiver, and then move the children on to other adults gradually once they have formed a steady attachment.

Join with the children. Rather than pointing out the attractions of the centre—that is, asking children to find what you offer interesting—instead, ask the children to bring in something from home that interests them and make an effort to become engaged with the children over whatever fascinates them. One suggestion provided to me recently was for a child to bring into the centre a compact disc that was being played in the car on the way, and play that until it ends. In this way, there is some continuity between home and the centre.

Explain exactly when the parent will return. Do not tell young children that 'Daddy will be back soon' when 'soon' can mean anything from a few minutes to a few hours (Greenman & Stonehouse 1997). Instead, explain that Dad will be back after a particular activity.

Accept children's feelings, even complaints about feeling ill, rather than telling them that it's all in their imagination. Comfort them when they are distressed, rather than trying to distract them from their feelings.

Make the children responsible for a solution. Having listened to children's concerns or ills, you could ask how they can help themselves to feel better. They might begin a favourite activity or ask one of the other children to play, for example. But if they are determined to remain miserable, you cannot prevent that.

Communicate your faith that they can cope. You can tell children that you know that they can find a way to feel happier. You might learn from the parents about other times when the children have overcome their feelings—such as being scared of the dark—and remind them of these occasions, expressing your faith that they can take charge of their feelings again.

Interrupt the pattern. In Chapter 10, pattern interruption was suggested as a solution to chronic problems. With respect to separation difficulties, this can mean changing the sequence of events. The usual sequence is that the parent and child arrive, the parent leaves, and the child becomes upset. It could help to rearrange this sequence so that the separation is less upsetting to everyone. For example, you could tell children that their parent is about to leave and they should become upset now, while their parent is still here to comfort them. Then, once they are calm, the parent can depart. If parents have inflexible working hours, this might require forward planning, such as arranging for them to arrive 15 minutes earlier for a week, so that there is time to provide their child with the comfort he or she requires.

The rationale for this suggestion is that when children have a long history of separation problems, they can become upset not so much that their parent is going, but that they feel so badly and are out of control of their distress. When children become hysterical, they need their parent—not a relative stranger—to reassure them.

Permit the crying. Normally, you will have tried to reassure distressed children that there is nothing to be upset about, tried to soothe their feelings and generally distract them from their distress. When this has not worked, you can instead instruct distressed children to cry, explaining that it is quite okay for sad children to cry. Find them a comfortable corner, tell them that you understand that they are sad and that they can be sad for as long as it takes: all day if necessary. If they stop crying, you can remind them that they do not have to stop if they still feel sad.

The rationale behind this suggestion is that children will continue to communicate their distress until someone says 'Message received'. Once they feel that others now understand, they do not need to keep letting you know how they feel. It also reflects the fact that, for some unknown reason, reassuring has not worked so, when something isn't working, you should stop doing it, as suggested in Chapter 10.

Check that children are not feeling responsible for their parent/s. Some children have taken on the job of looking after their parents, but they cannot perform this role unless they are with them, and so they refuse to separate. In my experience, this is most common to eldest children in large families who feel responsible for helping their parent with the younger siblings, youngest children who fear that their parent will be lonely if they are apart, and children whose parents are stressed (see Chapter 14).

This form of separation anxiety will not improve unless the children are convinced that their parent does not need them to look after her, and they can see the parents taking care of themselves. Even if stressed and not sure how they will solve their present problems, the parents need to reassure the child that they are working on finding a solution and are still available to look after the children in the family. It might be that you need to recommend some support agencies that can assist the family.

Recommend another placement. Centre-based child care does not suit every child. If individual children cannot settle at all in your centre even after patient and sensitive handling, it might be that a home environment (such as family day care) would suit their needs better. You might have to recommend this to their parents, in the interests of the children's emotional wellbeing.

Reunions

Even those children who separated reluctantly from their parents at the beginning of the day might be off-hand when their parents return to collect them. Ignoring the parents might simply reflect the fact that they were certain that their parents were going to return and are happy to stay on.

A second pattern is that some children resist going home. Greenman and Stonehouse (1997) explain that these reactions have nothing to do with the children's preferring to be in child care than home. Instead, their reluctance to leave can be an attempt to involve their parents in this important part of their lives.

Third, the children might see their parent and experience renewed sadness that they have been parted all day and so become distressed. This distress can be due to being exhausted and reacting when their defences are worn down.

When parents collect their children, suggest that they avoid telling them that they miss them, in case the children think that their parents need their company and so refuse to separate in future. Instead, they can tell their child that they are glad to see him or her, which is what they mean anyway.

Children who are picked up later often experience growing distress as they see other children going home before them. It can be useful to reserve some special activities for this time of the day and to make use of the improved adult-child ratio to give these children some special attention (Greenman & Stonehouse 1997).

Clinging to staff

There are many reasons why children might cling to an adult rather than becoming involved in the centre's activities:

- a child who is new to the centre might need some initial security before being confident enough to join in;

- a slow-to-warm-up child might need the same extra security, but for longer;
- the child's development might be out of step with the other children's. For example, children who are not steady on their feet can feel at risk of being knocked over by boisterous bigger children; or children whose development is advanced—that is, who are gifted—might have grown out of the activities that the other children are doing but cannot find an intellectual peer with whom they could play more sophisticated games;
- children's parents might have recently separated and now that they are being separated from their remaining parent, they are grieving or are frightened that they might lose that parent too; and
- the child might not know how to make friends.

Allocate a primary caregiver. Whatever the reason for clinging to staff, you can begin by allocating a primary caregiver for a period of time and giving children the extra attention they appear to need.

Mediate children's play. Help the children to begin a favourite activity and guide them to elaborate on their play. Then, once they are engaged, withdraw briefly and, over the course of a few weeks, gradually extend your absence.

Introduce other children gradually. You can draw in another child to be with the pair of you. Introduce the children to each other and tell them about an interest they have in common, even if it's simply that they are the same age. Make sure that reticent children do not just transfer their dependence from you to one other child by bringing in different children every now and then (Mitchell 1993).

Allocate tasks. You can give clingy children small tasks to do—perhaps first with you, then in parallel with you, and then on their own or in a pair with another child.

Extend the separation. Once they can move away from you for a short time, extend how long they are to manage without you by going off to another area to do something, while being sure to return within a negotiated time.

Teach social skills. If children cannot join in with the group because they lack the necessary social skills, try some of the suggestions in Chapters 5 and 12.

Use of manners

Children are more likely to say 'please' or 'thank you' if you do not praise or punish them when they do and don't. If you just respond to a thank you with,

'You're welcome' or something similar, children will naturally pick up these social graces.

If you want to insist that children say 'please' when requesting something, you could remind them to do so; when you want them to acknowledge that they are being given something, you could keep holding on to it until they say 'thank you'.

However, I do not insist every time because children have to ask for so many more things than adults do, and being chided constantly over their manners must become tiresome for them. Their manners will get more automatic over the years, and if you are willing to wait, your example will work its magic in time.

Transitions

Fields and Boesser (2002) say that making children wait is disrespectful: it wastes their time (as well as being an invitation to behavioural problems). This makes it important for you to manage transitions between activities so that the children who are ready early do not become restless while they await late-comers. It can help to:

- give warning of an impending change in activity so that the children can disengage in time;
- allow children to finish an activity in which they are engrossed, even if that means that they will have to start the new one late; and
- break the group into smaller groups for activities such as hand-washing.

Conclusion

The times when children are acquiring self-care skills are not routines to be rushed through in order to get to the 'real' curriculum: they are times to provide responsive care so that children learn that they are worth caring about (Greenman & Stonehouse 1997). Moreover, they are opportunities for children to practise many valuable skills—both content and process—and, in turn, to feel proud of their growing independence and competence. Therefore, although one purpose of routines will be to make these times manageable for caregivers, the main purpose is to make them enjoyable and achievable for the children. Disruptions that occur along the way need to be responded to with awareness that disturbances are inevitable given the demands of the tasks and the maturity of the children performing them.

12

●●

Social and play difficulties

> *Conflict is inevitable among members of any truly participatory group of children; it should not and probably cannot be eliminated completely. The spontaneous and inevitable social problems that arise when children work and play together put the teacher in an ideal position to advance children's social development.*

> KATZ AND MCCLELLAN (1997: 59)

Even when you can meet most children's needs most of the time, there will still be some occasions when children have social difficulties. Some of these come about because individual children lack a more mature skill or temporarily are overwhelmed emotionally and so cannot perform a skill that is within their repertoire; sometimes the behaviour—antisocial as it is—works for the child: it is quicker to snatch a toy than to ask for it. Sometimes, social and other behavioural difficulties come about because they have previously been responded to in controlling ways, in which case the behaviours are a reaction against these methods. In that case, these secondary behaviours will repair when a guidance approach replaces rewards and punishments.

The purpose of this chapter is to offer a range of suggestions for particular social difficulties that are common with young children. If you have already tried one of the ideas and have found that it has not worked in your particular situation, select another that might be useful.

Isolated children

There is a distinction between solitary play and reticence, whereby a child hovers on the outside of a group, appearing to be interested in joining the other children but not knowing how. Solitary play is likely to be positively beneficial for all children at some time during each day, but if reticence is prolonged, is associated with shyness or loneliness, it can be worthwhile for you to intervene.

Solitary play

All individuals of any age need some time to be alone: to rest, prepare for new situations, or observe those around them (Readdick 1993). Solitary play does not mean that preschool-aged children are failing to advance to the next stage of development: it is a normal part of any day.

Over the course of a day, children fluctuate in their ability to be sociable and their personalities differ too, so that some children need a lot of solitude while others are comfortable with being surrounded by people for much of the day. However, all children are more likely to tolerate having others around when there is enough space, when the group is a comfortable size, when there is a lot of opportunity to play in small groups, and when noise and temperature levels are reasonable.

Provide a withdrawal area. Because so much time in child care or preschool is shared with other children, it is important to provide a safe, inviting area in which individual children can be alone. This might be a window seat or a big chair with soft toys and quiet activities such as books or music.

Accept when children need to be by themselves. Forcing children to play with others when they do not want to could make them less rather than more willing to be sociable. Therefore, do not force children to take part in group activities, but instead aim to make these attractive enough to entice children out of their solitude (see Chapter 11).

Read children's behaviours that signal when they need to be alone. Children might signal that they need solitude by saying so, by creating territorial boundaries with their toys, by turning away from the other children and engaging in solitary play, or by withdrawing from the company of others (Readdick 1993). Children sometimes use aggression as a communication that they are not coping within a group. This can be handled as suggested in a later section.

Lonely children

Loneliness can come about when children have not yet located a friend or lose a friend through death or separation, or have changed neighbourhood or their care setting. Children who are suffering such losses will feel lonely, just as adults do, and they need the same understanding that lonely adults require. (See Chapter 14 for information on bereavement.)

Listen. Listen to lonely children and accept their feelings, even though you might feel distressed for them. Resist reassuring them that 'things are not so bad', as this tells them that they are not allowed to feel as they do. Instead, listening lets them know that you care about them and accept how they feel now.

Arrange soothing activities—such as water play—that are best done alongside or with other children. Once the children are comfortable with this parallel play, you could then introduce some cooperative games.

Children's books about the type of loss that lonely children are experiencing can be useful.

Match the child with peers. Sometimes children are lonely because there appears to be no one else in the group who is matched to them in terms of developmental levels or interests. If children are unaware of their common interests, you could mention these to them: 'Ahmed is interested in dinosaurs too, just like you. I wonder if you would like to play a dinosaur game together?'. Another strategy is to place children with atypical development in the company of their developmental rather than age peers (see Chapter 13).

Gain information from the children's parents about anything that might have happened at home to cause the loneliness, about what they suggest you could do to help their child, about what you are doing at the centre which they might want to support—say, by inviting one of the centre's children over to play—or suggesting books to read or outside professionals for the parents to consult if the child is having difficulties at home as well.

Make a referral. If the problem does not get better in the centre, together with the parents you might need to refer the child for help from other professionals.

Reticence (not joining in)

Sometimes, particular children do not manage to enter a group or develop friendships because they lack the necessary social skills. In turn, a lack of friendships means that the children do not have enough opportunity to practise and develop their social skills, and so the initial problem can grow. In the preschool years, shyness and withdrawal are not accurate predictors that children have or will develop social problems later, although young children will feel lonely when they are isolated and so reticence in young children is worth doing something about.

Deliver a program that is attractive, relevant and developmentally appropriate. Children will wander around aimlessly when their caregivers are not responding to their needs (Doherty-Derkowski 1995) or when the program does not interest them or match their developmental level. Therefore, check that your program is suitable for reticent children and respond appropriately and promptly when they are disengaged.

Assist children to enter a group. If children seem unable to negotiate entry into the play of other children, you could teach any of the social skills listed in Box 5.1 and use some of the other preventive measures listed in Chapter 5, such as ensuring that the children know each other's names. A more direct intervention is to structure an activity that involves just the reticent child and one other, then adding two, and then more as the reticent child becomes more comfortable.

Shyness

Whereas disruptive behaviour comes about because children are not monitoring their actions and thinking about these in advance, shy children monitor too much, worrying about the impression they are creating. Not everyone has to be outgoing, but shyness can be very painful and limiting to children, so it can be beneficial if they learn to overcome it.

Improve children's self-esteem. Use acknowledgment rather than praise to teach children not to rely on other people's opinions of them.

Normalise shyness. Acknowledge that we all feel unsure of ourselves (or shy) so it is normal. This removes the children's worry about being shy and so halves the problem.

Give children time to recover themselves. When young children become self-conscious as they all do, do not encourage this by calling it shyness ('Ooh, have you gone all shy?'). Instead, avoid comment and give them a moment or two to recover their self-possession.

Expect appropriate social behaviour. Expect children to greet others, but not necessarily when everyone is watching them. They might need a few minutes, after which they can approach you and say 'hello' less publicly. Insist, however, that they do so; otherwise the shyness will become an excuse for poor social skills. You can also advise children that no one will be able to tell if they are only pretending not to feel shy, compared with when they actually are not feeling shy. So they can pretend, and that will work.

Make children responsible for a solution. Talk with shy children about being boss of the shy feelings that sometimes overwhelm them. Just as other fears are a product of their imagination, fears about what others think of you are too, and so they will need to take charge of these thoughts. (See Chapter 9.)

Have fun. If nothing else has worked, you could prescribe the shyness—perhaps by telling shy children not to say 'hello' when they arrive at the centre, because you would get such a fright, or because they would not be able to cope. This exaggerates how silly the shyness is, making it obvious that nothing dreadful would happen if they overcame it.

Prejudice and discrimination

Some children reject others who look or behave unusually. This is not inevitable, however: children can be taught about differences between people in a way which conveys that differences are interesting, rather than deficiencies.

Prevention. Formulate a written anti-bias policy and supply this to all new parents when they enrol their child in your centre. You cannot demand that parents share your values, but they need to know what behaviours you will and will not condone in the centre.

Use books and natural events to talk with children about the differences between people (Crary 1992). The children's awareness of differences can be increased through inclusive wall displays or planned activities and discussions about how other people feel and live. However, this multi-cultural perspective should not degenerate into a 'tourist curriculum' which focuses on a culture's exotic customs rather than daily life, as that can perpetuate stereotypes (Derman-Sparks & the ABC Task Force 1989).

While bigotry assumes that differences mean that people are unequal, 'colour-blindness' assumes that differences do not matter (Stonehouse 1991b). Neither perspective is accurate. Instead, an anti-bias curriculum acknowledges and celebrates differences openly and honestly (Saifer et al. 1993) by giving children straightforward information about gender, race and ethnicity.

Prohibit the exclusion of other children. Establish general rules of using words that do not hurt other people (Derman-Sparks 1992) and of not excluding others from their play for reasons of race, gender, or disability (Derman-Sparks & the ABC Task Force 1989).

Mediate problem resolution. When an incident of teasing or verbal abuse has occurred, withdraw recipients and offenders together. Talk to *recipients* of the teasing: listen to them and say that you understand that what the other child said hurt their feelings. Meanwhile, allow the offender to hear this conversation, without being lectured to or shamed. When a child has not been humiliated, the teasing or abuse is more likely to stop.

As long as you can do so without preaching, give the perpetrator some simple information which clarifies a stereotype or misconception (Crary 1992).

Teach the victims to be assertive about teasing, using general statements such as, 'Don't say those things to me. I don't like it' or more specific rebuttals, such as, 'That is not friendly. I won't play with you if you're not friendly' or, 'That's not true. I'm not (whatever the other child accused him or her of being)'.

Give perpetrators opportunities to exercise power prosocially. Teasing can be some children's way of gaining power in situations where otherwise they feel powerless (Mitchell 1993), so ensure that perpetrators of discrimination feel accepted and powerful in your setting. Ensure that you offer many opportunities for choices and for making real contributions to the centre and that you acknowledge—but do not praise—children's achievements so that they learn how to value themselves and each other.

Exclusion

At times, a child or small group of children might refuse to let another child join their play, perhaps because of the child's devalued status, because they cannot absorb another player, or they want to be alone. Sometimes it is a form of bullying, where a group of children refuse their companionship as a way of hurting another child.

Clarify the reason. You can ask them about their play and whether there is room for one more child. Complaints such as, 'Matthew wants to be the baby and we already have a baby' could be met with suggestions that this family could have twins, or that Matthew could adopt some other role.

Negotiate delayed entry. If the children reject these suggestions, you could explain, 'Well, it looks like there isn't room for you in this game just now, Matthew. Children, how long do you think you'll be playing this game before you can let Matthew join in? How long will Matthew have to wait?'. This gives a certain end to their exclusion of Matthew and lets him know that it has to do with the demands of the game, rather than himself.

Support excluded children to be assertive. Teach vulnerable children to be assertive about their rights to play where and with whatever equipment they like. They have a right to a turn, which cannot be denied by others for an unreasonable period.

Prohibit bullying. Sometimes, a powerful member of a group draws other children into excluding a particular child with statements such as 'We don't want her to play with us, do we?' This is clearly an attempt to bully. In that case, you might draw on a previously established rule which states 'You can't say "you can't play",' and tell the perpetrator/s that the behaviour hurts the victim's feelings, and that it is not acceptable. If any or all of the children cannot consider this information and change how they are acting, this is a social tantrum (as defined in Chapter 6) and can be dealt with in any of the ways outlined in Chapter 9.

Aggression

Aggression is inconsiderate of the feelings of other children. Aggressive children's verbal and non-verbal behaviours often disrupt the play of other children with the result that they will have problems developing friendships. Therefore, you will need to respond to aggressive behaviour, both for the aggressors' own sake and to protect their peers.

Your aims when responding to aggression are to comfort the recipient; to teach aggressors another way to meet their needs and solve problems; and to reassure onlooking children about their ongoing safety—both from attacks on them by the perpetrator and from being dealt with harshly if they were to make a mistake by becoming aggressive. The basic premise is that non-violence is better than violence at solving problems (Slaby et al. 1995).

Prevention. Foster cohesion within the peer group, as aggression is less common within stable, cooperative groups (Farver 1996). Another preventive measure is to ensure that children are not crowded and competing for too few toys, as stress will make it more likely that they will use available toys as missiles or will snatch toys from each other.

A form of secondary prevention is to take action when a problem is brewing but the children are displaying only passive tantrums (see Chapter 6). As these often precede social aggression, you might be able to help children calm down before their feelings overwhelm them and lead to an aggressive outburst.

Build a close relationship with aggressive children. Their aggression can be exacerbated because their antisocial behaviour typically provokes rejection by their parents, educators and peers. Therefore, it is crucial that you do not allow their behaviour to provoke the same reaction in you (Kelly 1996). So it will be important that you take extra steps to build a close relationship with aggressive children to compensate for their lack of attachments to peers and other adults.

Check the children's language skills. In my experience, many children are aggressive habitually when they lack the requisite language skills to communicate with others or to direct their own actions. Therefore, if individual children's language abilities seem a likely cause of their aggression, seek parental permission for a speech pathology assessment.

Teach prosocial skills. Toddlers who act aggressively or who bite might need guidance about how instead to use words to express what they want. Older children might need coaching in how to enter a group without disrupting its ongoing activity (Kelly 1996)—see Chapter 5. As aggressive children are more likely to interpret their peers' accidental behaviours as intentionally hostile and subsequently respond aggressively, some may need coaching to make more accurate interpretations of others' intent and to overlook occasional mistakes by playmates (Asher 1983; Katsurada & Sugawara 1998).

Keep in mind, however, that aggressive children tend to associate with others of a similar nature, in which case you will need to coach all members of an aggressive clique so that all improve their behaviour (Farver 1996).

Teach aggressive children to manage their emotions. Aggressive children might already know how to act prosocially but lack the self-control to enact these behaviours, in which case they do not need more information but require guidance to learn self-control, in ways recommended in Chapter 9.

Support victims. Teach recipients of aggression how to negotiate with rather than to reject the aggressor, so that peer rejection does not provoke further outbursts of violence (Arnold et al. 1999). Allow recipients of aggression some time to be assertive independently to establish their own place in the group hierarchy (Farver 1996) but if safety becomes an issue or resolution is not speedy, step in to protect recipients from further intimidation (Arnold et al. 1999).

Use time away for perpetrators if necessary—but not as a punishment, simply as recognition that their behaviour tells you that they cannot play in a friendly way at the moment. Once they are calm again, you might have to help them to engage in a new activity (Slaby et al. 1995).

Give aggressors alternative opportunities to lead and exercise autonomy rather than trying to exert control in destructive ways.

Educate children about the effects on recipients. Babies are sometimes accused of playing aggressively when their actions are just a developmentally clumsy attempt to touch and explore. In these instances, you can show them how to touch gently or point out that the recipient is not enjoying how he or she is being touched. The babies will not necessarily understand your words but will realise that they are being given an explanation and so will not persist in a secondary reaction against a prohibition. You could also attract the perpetrator's interest to an alternative activity.

With older children, your education about the effects of the behaviour can coincide with soothing the victim. Take the perpetrator and victim aside and address the victim, not the perpetrator, reflecting the victim's feelings: 'That hurt you, didn't it? . . . Yes, Shelley forgot to use her words . . . She might be feeling frustrated or angry, do you think?'.

Next, nurse the recipient's injuries and invite (but do not force) those who inflicted them to help, so that they are encouraged to be responsible for their actions. Meanwhile, do not require perpetrators to apologise. If you shame them into doing so, you might provoke another incident. Instead, you might apologise on their behalf. 'I know when Shelley calms down, she will feel very sorry to have hurt you. I'm sure she will want to say sorry then, but I will say it for her now. I am sorry that she hurt you'. This validates the victim's hurt feelings without confronting perpetrators with their mistakes.

If necessary, you could later explain to perpetrators briefly, and without anger what effect the aggression had, as long as you can do so without humiliating them. However, keep these explanations brief because aggressive children are likely to have heard it all before. Aggression usually results from a lack of self-control rather than a lack of information about prosocial behaviour, so giving more information is pointless.

Shadow children who are habitually aggressive (see Chapter 8), so that you can observe their behaviour with the aim of identifying its triggers or signs of passive tantrums that might precede aggressive behaviour. Meanwhile, your presence can lend support for them to regain command of their emotions and thus avoid further outbursts.

Acknowledge prosocial acts. When you observe that children who are frequently aggressive are instead behaving prosocially, acknowledge that you (and their playmate) appreciate it. Remember not to praise, though, for the reasons discussed in Chapter 2.

Support the parents of perpetrators. Where possible, support parents of aggressive children to improve their bond with their children by using a guidance approach to discipline. This will give the children experience of empathy and nurturance and allow them to learn how to be empathic towards others.

You could also encourage parents to provide additional opportunities for the children to practise prosocial skills in relationships with family acquaintances or other children from the centre (Hartup & Moore 1990).

Inform the victim's parents. Without telling the victim's parents the name of the perpetrator, notify the parents of both children about the incident. However, make it clear that you have sorted it out and that you do not expect the parents to solve it for you. You do not want the perpetrator punished at home for something that has happened at the centre. Your rationale for informing parents is simply that they have a right to know about their child's behaviour or injuries.

Refer to specialists. If individual children do not respond to the above methods, you will need to suggest to their parents that they consult a specialist in children's behaviour. If they are unwilling to do this and your disciplinary efforts ultimately prove unsuccessful, you might have to consider asking the parents to withdraw their child from the centre, in the interests of keeping the other children safe. This sounds harsh but might be therapeutic in that it could shock the parents into helping their child; it also protects the other children, who have a right to feel safe in your care. (If the economics of losing an enrolment concern you, keep in mind that if the problem is not resolved, you could end up losing more than one of the victims, which would have even greater cost implications for the centre.)

Biting

Biting is like any other aggressive behaviour that hurts or injures a child's playmates. The same preventive measures are relevant, and intervening with older toddlers and young children can be similar to the measures for other types of aggression.

With babies, however, intervention can have some added dimensions. Sometimes, quite without malice, under-one-year-olds bite another child who happens to be there. Babies put things in their mouths, and that 'thing' can occasionally be another child. You can respond as follows.

- Check that the baby is not uncomfortable in the mouth because of teething. Administer medication such as paracetamol for acute pain, and offer teething rings to soothe low-grade pain.
- You might choose to say 'No' or 'Stop' firmly to a baby who has bitten. (I reserve the word 'No' for dangerous behaviour, and avoid it for simple mistakes.)
- Offer the child something else to bite or eat, explaining, 'Teeth are for eating. Here is something you can eat' (Mitchell 1993); and
- Avoid large group activities, and avoid placing a repeated biter with his or her favourite victim (Greenman & Stonehouse 1997).

Rough-and-tumble play

Some children use rough-and-tumble play as a way of inviting another child to play with them. They do not mean to be aggressive, but they might not notice the other child's protests. In these cases, you can:

- remind children to use words when they want to invite another child to play;
- when appropriate, provide a mat for tumbling and other physically active games, and lead cooperative games that allow children to touch each other safely; and
- explain how the other child is feeling about unwanted touch. If, after these reminders, the instigators of rough play do not change their behaviour, this is no longer a social problem, but a loss of self-control. It can be dealt with as described in Chapter 9.

Super-hero play

When TV programs with themes of power and subordination become popular, some children will carry over the violent themes into their play at the centre. Super-hero play can help children work out issues of good and evil and power and powerlessness (Saifer et al. 1993). Or, the play can simply be an imitation of what they have seen, in which case it is merely ritualistic and does not help children make sense of their world (Gronlund 1992).

Dawkins (1991) suggests that we cannot ban violent play in early childhood centres because it helps children to understand their world. She believes also that children need an exciting environment which is full of adventure, challenge and exploration.

On the other hand, violent play has some significant disadvantages. First, it can mean that children whose play is often violent are not experimenting enough with their play themes as they concentrate almost exclusively on their super-hero play. Second, super-hero play can deteriorate quickly into outright aggression (Gronlund 1992). Third, children who were not originally involved in the violent play can imitate the other children's aggression both at the time and later—although this effect mostly occurs for children who were already aggressive (Dawkins 1991). Fourth, the violence of the play can intimidate the children who are observing it. Fifth, victims of the make-believe violence usually do not enjoy it (Bergen 1994). These disadvantages give rise to the following suggestions for limiting the potential negative effects of play that has violent themes.

Give children other opportunities to resolve issues of power and

powerlessness. Give children opportunities to make choices and take responsibility so that they are powerful in their own lives. This avoids the need to use dramatic play to resolve issues of powerlessness. In so doing, ensure that girls as well as boys can participate in the games and discussions about power and safety. Boys may be the main instigators of games with powerful themes, but girls need to participate as well so that they become aware of their own power.

Within your curriculum, explore issues of power and safety by using alternative topics such as dinosaurs, space adventures, or nightmares. Protectiveness training can also address safety issues for young children.

Become familiar with the programs so that you understand their attraction for the children (Cupit 1989) and so you can incorporate their themes into your educational program and, in so doing, moderate any negative effects the programs can have on the children (Dawkins 1991).

Let the children teach you about their heroes so that you can share rather than disparage their interests (Gronlund 1992). This communicates that you accept their experiences and feelings, allows you to ask questions that help them to be critical of what they see on TV, gives you credibility when you discuss aggression with them, and ensures that their play does not become surreptitious. More important, however, it allows you to provide support for the children as they work out scary feelings and reach their own conclusions about hurting other people (Gronlund 1992).

Redirect the play. Have available a range of attractive dramatic play materials that can encourage the children to play other games as well as their favourite super-hero games. Ensure that there is enough time and equipment for gross physical activity, so that the more active children are able to use their energies without needing to play the super-hero games exclusively.

You might offer cooperative activities to balance the largely competitive themes of super-hero play. Or, you could provide alternative game scenarios that do not involve violence but which still give children power (Saifer et al. 1993). For example, you could move the danger source from a person to an event, and have the children conquer the danger—for example, by tracking down a wild animal or putting out a fire.

Restrict the play. You could cordon off a section of the outside play area in which the super-hero play is permitted, so that the remaining area feels safe to the other children. Another form of restriction is to insist that the play has to be pretend play, and that no one is to get hurt. Gronlund (1992) recommends teaching children that on TV, the real actors use stunt-men and -women who practise the moves carefully to ensure that no one gets hurt, and so the children also need to practise making the moves safely.

Alternatively, you could set a time limit on the super-hero play. It might be easier to use natural changes of routine—such as fruit time—as a signal to stop the play and settle into a new activity.

Finally, you can check with participating children that they still want to play the game. It is important to suspend the game if any of the children are not feeling safe (Bergen 1994).

Extend the play. Help the children to extend their super-hero play scenarios into more positive themes. You can begin with their script but add new parts and new conclusions that are more positive (Gronlund 1992). This avoids the play being a simple repetition of someone else's script and so teaches children dramatic play skills.

Teach critical skills. If you watch TV or videotapes within your session, you can teach the children to be active viewers rather than passive recipients of what they see. Once they have learned to evaluate what they see on TV, they can begin to make judgments about the violent programs they are copying in their play (Dawkins 1991).

Enlist parental support. Finally, it can be useful to talk with parents whose children do not seem to be growing out of the super-hero phase. The parents might not know that their children are obsessed with the violence and, once aware of the issue, might decide to limit their TV viewing. It can also be useful to encourage parents to buy open-ended toys that allow for creative play rather than TV-related toys that have only one purpose (Gronlund 1992).

Unwillingness to share

It strikes me that we often expect children to be better at sharing than we adults are. Just like us, children need some territory that is theirs alone and they have the right to choose with whom to share. With this said, some ways of promoting sharing include the following.

Prevent disputes. Have available enough toys to avoid repeated disputes over equipment. Ensure that there are enough attractive alternatives so that a child is just as happy with one item as with another. Meanwhile, it might be useful to ask children to bring to the centre only those personal toys that they are happy for other children to touch. (The exception will be soft toys for sleep time and which children do not have to share.)

Give children permission to finish playing with a toy before being expected to hand it over to another child. This allows them some control over sharing, which increases the likelihood that they will be happy to share appropriately.

Structure turn-taking. When children are having to wait for turns on equipment, an egg timer can help them to be aware of the passage of time. Or, you can have the children write their name on a 'waiting list' so that they do not have to hover idly near the desired equipment, which wastes their time and puts pressure on the children who are using the equipment to defend their place. If the children are too young to write their name, you could have each child's name written on a small card with a velcro dot attached to its back. They can find their name card and stick it to a waiting list board equipped with velcro patches.

On the other hand, you do not want to be overseeing these arrangements completely. Help the children to be responsible for negotiating turn-taking, or else you will have to be judge and jury in a constant stream of disputes and will be asked to respond to repeated cries of, 'It's not fair!'.

Explain non-judgmentally that it is friendly to share toys with your friends, and also acknowledge or thank (but do not praise) children for being friendly when they have shared with another child.

Encourage restitution. When a baby has snatched a toy from another child and the other is not protesting, ignore this (Greenman & Stonehouse 1997). If the other baby is protesting, see if you can help them both to find a toy that interests them. When older children have snatched a toy from another child, you could give them a restricted choice, for example: 'You can give that back to Tim, or you can put it down over there'. This allows the perpetrator to save face while still returning the contested item.

Support bereaved children. Children who have suffered a profound emotional deprivation such as the loss of a parent through a death or separation, tend to be less able to share and often hoard items that they do not even require. It's as if they have learned early to grasp anything that's going, because they never know when it will not be there any more. It could help to let them bring some precious items to the centre without having to share them, to support them in their grieving (see Chapter 14), and to use disciplining techniques that are firm but gentle, so that the children gain confidence emotionally in the adults who remain caring for them.

Avoid being moralistic about stealing. Some children take home or hide items that are not theirs, in order to avoid having to share these. In response, you could explain that the centre needs all of its toys so that there is something for the children to play with, or that another child will miss a personal item if it is lost. As young children do not fully comprehend ownership and sharing, treat this not as a misbehaviour—that is, do not call it stealing—but as a lack of knowledge on the child's part.

Telling tales

Children will often approach you with a description of what another child is doing wrong. Telling tales usually comes about because of normal development: young children go through a natural stage of having too much respect for rules and they cannot yet distinguish important rules (those that ensure safety) from other less crucial ones. So, they report everything, are told off for doing so, and then are chastised when they do not report dangerous behaviour.

Telling tales can also come about when adults rely heavily on rewards and punishments in their discipline. With only so many 'goodies' (so much approval) to go around, the children will compete with each other for the most. From the children's perspective, this means making another child look bad so that they can look good in comparison.

With this information as a background, some strategies for dealing with telling tales include the following.

Teach children to discriminate between safety and other issues. Involve verbal children in formulating behavioural guidelines so that, in this process, they learn the reasons for rules and can eventually learn to distinguish important rules from the less crucial ones. Explain that it is vital to tell if there is danger, but not otherwise. Children who tell tales might simply be noticing behaviour that is not allowed at home and are assuming that it is not allowed at the centre either (Mitchell 1993). In this case, you could explain that it is not a problem because it is not hurting anyone and is safe. Children are able to adjust to different rules in different settings and so usually will cope with this.

Encourage assertiveness. Encourage children to tell a rule-breaker that they do not like the behaviour. Teach them that if they have done this and the offender has not desisted, they can come to you and ask for your *help* to get the child to stop. In this way, they are not coming to tell tales, but are letting you know they need assistance.

Suggest positive tale-telling. If individual children continue to tell you whenever another child does not live up to their expectations, you could encourage them to notice positive things that the other children do and report those to you instead (Mitchell 1993).

Do not punish children who have broken a rule. Punishments create competition between children, lowering their self-esteem and encouraging them to tell on each other so that the tale-bearer looks good by pointing out what another child is doing wrong.

Restrict children's responsibilities. Never make young children responsible for supervising another child. This can teach them to tell tales out of fear of under-reporting something serious. They are not yet mature enough to judge what is serious and what is not.

Finally, if children report something that you have already noticed or identify a culprit when you're more interested in a solution, you can thank them briefly and let them know that you will deal with it (Mitchell 1993).

Packing away equipment

Planning how to tidy up a whole area of toys in logical steps can be too difficult for youngsters to do without help. (It's like having to tidy up the kitchen the morning after a party.) The following are some suggestions that could help children to participate in tidying up after an activity.

Assist with planning. Help the children to plan how to go about tidying up, or ask if they would like some suggestions.

Turn packing away into a game. Turn tidying up into a game that helps organise the task, for example, 'Simon says, put away everything that's red . . . and now, everything that has wheels' and so on.

Help children to tidy up. Like most activities that children do, they are happiest performing them when they have some company so participate in the packing away yourself, as they will be more likely to accompany you.

Give them a day off. If individual children generally help to pack away and today's refusal is uncommon, give them a day off. Let them know that you appreciate that they usually help and that everyone needs a day off sometimes, and express your faith that they will feel like helping next time.

Treat it as a passive tantrum. If children's refusal to assist with packing away is just one of many uncooperative behaviours, you could treat that as a passive tantrum and deal with it as recommended in Chapter 9.

Exploration of genitals

As babies are soothed and cared for physically, become increasingly mobile, and acquire toileting control, they are learning about and delighting in their bodies (Klass 1999). Once they are able to remove their own clothes and their arms grow long enough to reach the end of their trunk, they will inevitably discover the extra sensitivity of their genitals. However, Klass asserts that it is a mistake to think of touching the genital area as 'masturbation' as children do not experience adult-like sexual pleasure from such explorations.

Some will use genital touching to calm themselves. As this is normal, it can be responded to with acceptance, although you might suggest doing it in private. However, if children are engaging in this form of self-calming excessively, it could be worth exploring whether they are unduly stressed or to provide alternative sensory activities to calm them (see Soden 2002a, 2002b). And if they attempt to engage other children in sexualised play, it is likely that this is being imposed on them—that is, they are being sexually abused—in which case, a referral to a child welfare agency is called for.

Fears

Some children say that they are frightened of a variety of inoffensive objects—such as balloons, the sound of a toilet flushing, the sound of the hand drier, or going outside. As these fears restrict their activities and social inclusion, intervention is required. The following are some possible methods for doing this.

Listen. First, listen to children talk about their fears. If there is a good reason for their fear, try to remove its source. Understand that they are fearful even if you do not agree that the fear is warranted. But even if the fear seems ridiculous, do not tell them to 'stop being silly'. If you tell children that they are not allowed to be frightened, they will become frightened that no one will help them, and worried that they will not be able to hide their fear from others. These two feelings make the original problem worse than it was.

Take the panic out of being afraid. Normalise what they are feeling. You might explain that everyone gets frightened at times, or you can teach them the difference between being frightened of something, versus disliking it, versus being surprised by it. Sometimes we appear to be afraid of a cockroach, say, when we really have been surprised to find it somewhere unexpectedly. Being surprised or disliking something is not as scary as being frightened of it.

Have faith that they can overcome their fears. Armed with information from their parents, tell children stories about other times they have overcome problems, and express your confidence that they can do so again. Let them know that you think they are very brave for trying to be boss of their fears.

Make them responsible for a solution. Ask children how they plan to overcome their fears. As these are a product of the children's imagination, only they can change their thinking. You might explain that their fears are sneaking up on them and that children who are growing up on the inside as well as the outside will find a way to out-sneak them. Once they have decided to become boss of their fears, you could offer to be their 'fears adviser'. You know about magic spells that can get rid of fears, and they know about their own brain and so, because young children believe in magic, together you could invent a magic spell that will make the fears go away.

Copying disruptive behaviour

Sometimes, children will copy the silly behaviour of a friend. This is normal and so it can take the heat out of the situation by simply clicking your tongue in mock annoyance and saying something like, 'Four year olds! Still, at your age, you need times when you can have fun and be silly. Looks like this is one of those times'. Another thing you can do is point out quietly that humour arises when something is unexpected and so, once people can predict the behaviour, it stops being funny. You might say that it's fun to be silly, as long as it does not go on for too long. If you find that it is starting to impinge on other children or yourself, you can be assertive about the behaviour.

Conclusion

Early childhood is an ideal time for assisting children to act prosocially, as they are inherently motivated to socialise with other children and because there are many natural occasions during their play when you can guide their behaviour. In most cases, your guidance will allow the children to acquire the skills they need to develop companionable relationships.

Suggested further reading

The following titles examine many issues pertaining to an anti-bias curriculum, with some containing extensive lists of children's and adults' books on this theme:

Dau, E. (Ed.) (2001). *The anti-bias approach in early childhood*. (2nd ed.) Sydney: Addison-Wesley.

Derman-Sparks, L. & the A.B.C. Task Force (1989). *Antibias curriculum: Tools for empowering young children*. Washington, DC: National Association for the Education of Young Children.

Stonehouse, A. (1991). *Opening the doors: Child care in a multi-cultural society*. Watson, ACT: Australian Early Childhood Association.

Thompson, B.J. (1993). *Words can hurt you: Beginning a program of anti-bias education*. Menlo Park, CA: Addison-Wesley.

For promotion of pro-social behaviour, you might like to refer to:

Katz, L.G. & McClellan, D.E. (1997). *Fostering children's social competence: The teacher's role*. Washington, DC: National Association for the Education of Young Children.

Slaby, R.G., Roedell, W.C., Arezzo, D. & Hendrix, K. (1995). *Early violence prevention: Tools for teachers of young children*. Washington, DC: National Association for the Education of Young Children.

13

●●

Developmental challenges

> The aim of early intervention is to optimise children's learning
> by making use of their strengths and attempting to circumvent
> their difficulties to improve their daily functioning and wellbeing
> (Cook et al. 2000). It also aims at supporting families in their
> role of meeting their child's needs.
>
> Porter (2002a, 2002b: 4)

Very young children will naturally lack the skills of their older counterparts. As this is well understood by adults, the children's lack of skilfulness is seldom regarded as a behavioural difficulty. However, some older children do not acquire the skills expected for their age, which is manifested as developmental delays and is sometimes accompanied by behaviour patterns that are typical of younger children.

Speech and language skills

Comprehension or *language* skills refer to how much children can understand; *speech* refers to what ideas children can express; while *articulation* refers to how clearly they can form speech sounds. Obviously, articulation delays have social implications as they can impair others' understanding of children's speech. Also articulation errors can have causes (such as poor awareness of the sounds of language) that will affect the children's progress in other domains such as reading. Meanwhile, speech or language difficulties clearly restrict children's ability to converse with others but, perhaps even more importantly, limit their ability to talk to themselves about their own behaviour. This can lead to a range of behavioural difficulties—such as aggression that arises through frustration or the inability to use language to solve disputes—and even some less evident problems with the likes of toilet training (as the children cannot talk to themselves about the sensations that signal the need to go to the toilet); packing away toys (which has to be planned in logical steps through self-talk); and impulse control, as the children cannot talk to themselves about potential outcomes of their actions.

Children can experience *delays* in language, speech or articulation. Or, their development might occur out of the usual sequence or order—in which case this is described as 'disordered' or *impaired*. Children with delayed speech or language are relatively easy to identify when you have same-aged children with whom to compare them and when you are aware of the normal developmental milestones. (Most of us need to refer to our favourite checklist for these.) However, disordered or impaired speech or language can be difficult to detect. The children might understand some complex language and yet confuse easier concepts or can appear to be using language appropriately—such as asking, 'What you doing?' while you are preparing a snack—but they do not absorb the answer or appear to notice that you have answered them. There would be other signs of language impairment, such as a delay in speaking, poor attention to words, and difficulty with comprehension.

Language skills are absolutely crucial for children's ongoing cognitive development and for forming friendships. The longer speech or language difficulties go unchecked, the more areas of their development become affected. Therefore, it is crucial to talk early with parents if their child appears to have difficulties with speech or language. With their permission, it can be useful to seek specialist advice and to ensure that the child's hearing has been checked.

Not following directives

Children can usually understand sentences that are two or three words longer than the sentences they speak. If you exceed this, they can appear to be uncooperative when in fact they simply have not understood what you were asking them to do.

Simplify your instructions. To help, you can simplify what you say. For instance, if you tell children with language difficulties that there will be cake for afternoon tea, they will hear the word 'cake' and think that you are offering it now. Disappointment and confusion will arise when it does not appear immediately.

In the same vein, keep your instructions to one or two parts. Rather than saying, 'I want you to go to your bag, get your teddy and lie down', you could say, 'Time to get teddy and lie down'. If you add extra words into your instruction, children sometimes remember only the first thing you said, and so might go to their bag, forget what they were there to retrieve, wander off and then get chastised for not following instructions.

Check that the children have understood. Once children have verbal skills, you can ask them to repeat back what you have just said so that you are sure that they have understood.

Help them to cooperate. If they cannot translate what you are saying into an action, help them to get started. Guide them to where they need to be and initiate the physical action—such as picking up a block and dropping it in its container. If with these physical cues, the children still cannot cooperate, treat that as a refusal rather than an inability—and use the strategies mentioned in Chapter 9 for helping children get in command of their feelings so that they can follow even those directives that they find distasteful.

Refusal to talk (elective mutism)

Some children refuse for months to speak in a particular setting such as at preschool, whereas in other places they talk freely. Unlike most childhood behavioural difficulties, their refusal to talk in safe environments represents over—as opposed to under—control of their behaviour. Elective mutism can delay children's development as it restricts their participation, isolates them from other people, and channels their energies away from learning into exercising such restrictive self-control. So, some strategies to encourage silent children to talk include the following.

Take them out of the spotlight. When children first enter a room, we often put them under a social spotlight: everyone watches them. Under this public glare, it can be more difficult for them to talk, so let them know that it is okay not to greet you right away, but encourage them to say hello later when others are no longer watching.

Gentle teasing. If taking the pressure off does not help, you can try teasing them out of their silence by instructing them not to talk to you as you'd be so shocked you'd probably fall over in a faint, and then what would they do?

Indirect communication. A next step if this fails is to have them talk through a toy—perhaps a doll, teddy, or hand puppet—to your equivalent toy.

Let them save face. To ensure that children who have been refusing to speak do not lose face by starting to talk, you could sit back to back with them and let them talk to you less directly, or you could ask them to whisper or sing what they want to say, so that they can talk (which is your aim) but on their own terms.

Allow them to retain their cultural language. Sometimes I have met bicultural children who refuse to use English even when they know it, out of loyalty to their parents and the language everyone speaks at home. You might ask the parents if they can reassure their child that they are happy for him or her to use both languages.

Articulation errors

Many children of preschool age are still not yet accurate with saying the single sounds: th, r, l, sh, ch and s; and have difficulty with blends containing r, l, and s (such as 'tree', 'play' and 'spoon'). Difficulties will also depend on whether the sounds come in the beginning, middle or end of a word. Multi-syllabic words (such as animal, hospital, and ambulance) are often still difficult for children who are nearing school age. Most substitutions for these sounds are developmentally normal; others indicate a speech difficulty. If in doubt, ask parents for permission to refer their child to a speech pathologist.

Accept approximations. When young children are learning to talk, do not point out their articulation errors; instead, simply model the correct sound. For instance, when a child has called a cat a 'tat', you can respond positively with, 'Yes, that's a cat'. Young children will hear the difference and learn how to say the word correctly. In the meantime, do not try to force them to say it properly. That will come. Similarly, when they make grammatical mistakes such as using 'runned' instead of 'ran', you might naturally be able to use the correct form yourself without naming the error: 'Yes—he ran across the playground, didn't he? I saw him too'.

If difficulties continue, refer for a speech pathology assessment. If children's articulation errors do not improve and these make it difficult for other people to understand them at an age when you would expect their speech to be getting quite clear, it will be useful to request their parents' permission for a review by a speech pathologist. If intervention proves necessary, this can prevent children from becoming frustrated and it will avoid social difficulties that can arise when other people do not understand them. Sometimes, children's speech is unclear because they do not discriminate the sounds that make up the language (which is called 'phonological awareness') and if they cannot discern the sounds, they will have trouble learning to read. It is far more successful to treat this problem before school age than after.

Baby talk

Four-year-olds often like to revert to baby talk. They enjoy playing with their voices and finding out what sounds they can make. They will also chant, experimenting with rhyme and rhythms. This is necessary for their language development so should not be discouraged. However, if it becomes intrusive, you could use empathic assertion, as in: 'I know that it's fun to play with your voices and with words. But it will be time to find another game soon as the noise is bothering those of us playing over here'.

Asking repeated questions

Children learn how to make statements before they learn how to ask questions. But once they have mastered the question format, they realise that asking one gets you to speak to them, even if they already know the answer. This can be fine for a while, but the twentieth 'Why?' can be irritating.

Answer once or twice. You could answer the same question just once or twice, or ask children what they think the answer is.

Teach them to notice when to stop. When you are tired of the subject, you could tell them that you need some time now for your own thoughts, so that they learn to discriminate when it's time for asking questions and time to be quiet.

Have some fun. If all else fails, tickle the children until they cannot ask any more questions. Ask if they think their questions are all tickled out.

Check their comprehension levels. Check that children do not have a language impairment, as this can cause them to ask repeated questions that seem appropriate to the activity, but which are really just something they have learned to say in that situation and they do not appreciate that they are asking for or being given some information.

Telling lies

Children under four might say things that you think are a lie, but are really just fantasies or wishes. Later on (nearer the age of five), children will tell lies to get themselves out of trouble and to deny guilt. Sometimes, though, they only mean to say that they did it, but did not mean it to turn out so badly.

Expand on wishes. You can handle children's 'tall stories' by going along with and extending the fantasy.

Teach the difference between wishes and reality. You can ask gently or playfully whether what they are saying is a wish or hope. It takes a few years for children to distinguish fact from fantasy, and in the meantime you can guide them about the difference.

Do not demand confessions. Look for solutions to problems rather than culprits, so do not ask who performed a misdeed: set about finding a solution.

Respond fairly. Children tell lies to get themselves out of trouble. But if you do not punish them for misdeeds, there is no trouble to avoid and so they are more likely to confess an error when asked. When you react reasonably and predictably to mistakes, next time they will not anticipate an uncertain or harsh reprisal following an admission of responsibility.

Expressing anger at adults

Children will often say that they hate you when they actually mean that they are angry. They do this because they do not have many words to describe their feelings.

Reflect the anger. To respond to children's expressions of hate, you can say, 'You're angry at me at the moment' or you might even reflect the first feeling that caused them to be angry—namely, being hurt or disappointed. In this way, you are expanding their vocabulary of feeling words.

Help them to regain their composure. Often, listening is enough to tell them that what they feel is okay. If they seem to need help to calm down again, you could ask them what they can do to make themselves feel better.

Resist inflicting guilt. Resist the temptation to tell angry children that you still love them as this might cause them to feel guilty for being angry at you. In the early childhood years, children can feel only one emotion at a time (Kostelnick et al. 1998) and so are unaware in the heat of the moment that they also like you as well as being angry with you. Likewise, this is not the time to say that you love them but do not like their behaviour, because that is a difficult concept for young children to grasp, particularly in times of stress. Because they can feel emotions only in sequence rather than in combination, they are unaware that *you* can feel split emotions to the same event.

'Answering back'

If you find that children 'answer back' when you tell them off, or that they use a tone of voice that you think is 'cheeky', this could mean that you are using controlling discipline approaches, and the children are rebelling against these. In other words, this is a secondary behavioural problem, rather than something being instigated by the children's personality. When your own tone of voice is courteous and you try to lead rather than boss children, they will usually treat you with the same respect in return.

Use active ignoring. If they continue with a disrespectful tone of voice, you could let them know that you will not respond to them until they speak to you more respectfully (in a 'nicer' way).

Be assertive. You can be assertive when you find their tone of voice offensive.

Treat it as a social tantrum. If they persist in being disrespectful, treat that as a sign that they are out of control of their feelings—that is, they are in the midst of a social (verbal) tantrum and need your help to get back in control of themselves (see Chapter 9).

Swearing

There are three forms of swearing: swearing at someone; using swear words in place of adjectives; and swearing in frustration. The first is verbal abuse and is a sign that individuals are out of control of their feelings and need to be dealt with accordingly (see Chapter 9); the second and third types might respond to the following measures.

Ignore first occasions. The first time you hear an offensive word, it can pay to ignore it. You might let the child know that you are doing so.

Permit chanting. Almost all four-year-olds go through a stage of chanting—and will choose swear words so that they can experience what it feels like to be a bit wicked. (They go through this again at the age of eight in the form of poo and bum jokes.) Because this is so normal, you might decide to tolerate it for a while, but to let them know when it stops being funny.

Pretend to complain. I find it useful to do some mock complaining about children's fascination with wicked words: 'Oh no! Do I have to put up with this for a whole year, do I? Can I run away until it stops?'. This accepts that all children play with language and recognises that it doesn't harm anyone.

Be assertive. If you find their language really offensive, or if you are concerned that surrounding children might copy their language, you could:

- tell the children that someone has taught them the wrong words to a song they are chanting, and that you'll teach them the right ones;
- assert your rights: 'I don't like to hear words like that'. (If the children argue that other people use these words, you can simply state that other people might not mind them, whereas you do, and you have a right to ask them to respect your needs); and
- explain that the parents of surrounding children might not like those words and so if other children copied them, that could get them into trouble at home.

Expand their vocabulary. You might ask children if they know what the word means and say that it's better not to use words we don't understand. You could replace the swear word with another, more interesting word: for example, when they tell you about a 'bloody big dog' you can agree that, yes, it's enormous.

Avoid punishment. Punishing children will not stop them swearing: instead, they will repeat the words under their breath to prove that they can get away with it and you cannot stop them. Keep your faith that the above measures will suffice.

The attention deficit disorders

There are two types of attention-deficit disorders: ADHD which comprises inattentiveness *and* hyperactivity (verbal and/or physical); and ADD which involves inattentiveness only. The terms are relatively new labels for a condition which was first identified a hundred years ago and which has variously been described as hyperactivity, minimal brain dysfunction and hyperkinesis (Anastopoulos & Barkley 1992).

Although ADD is more prevalent, ADHD is referred to specialists more often (Hinshaw 2000). Most estimates say that around 3% to 5% of children and adolescents have ADHD (Wodrich 1994), with little variation across socioeconomic groups and with more boys than girls being recognised. Most children show their first signs of the conditions at between three and four years of age and, to be diagnosed, must have evidenced the symptoms prior to the age of seven years (Anastopoulos & Barkley 1992).

In the early childhood years in particular, it is difficult to distinguish normal childhood exuberance from ADHD, making accurate diagnosis difficult. Diagnosis is also complicated by the fact that the children's behaviour varies according to the circumstances and that their attention skills can be deficient in different ways—such as coming to attention, versus attention span.

Some writers believe that impulsivity is at the heart in particular of the hyperactive and combined forms of the disorders. In turn, this leads to a lack of emotional regulation, poor judgment, lack of organisational skills, problems with self-monitoring, a high rate of accidental injuries, impaired relationships with peers and family, emotional difficulties including depression and anxiety, and learning difficulties such as poor phonological awareness (despite having average intellectual abilities overall) (Hinshaw 2000). These children have a higher than usual rate of health problems such as incoordination, sleep disturbances, middle ear and upper respiratory infections, asthma, and allergies (Anastopoulos & Barkley 1992).

The cause of the attention deficit disorders is not known. Those who take a biological (as opposed to an environmental) view of the conditions contend that the behaviours are due to immaturity in how the frontal parts of the brain function. This area of the brain is responsible for planning and impulse control. However, the cause of this apparent neurological immaturity is not clear—although genetics, family environment, or the mother's health during pregnancy have all been implicated (Anastopoulos & Barkley 1992; Barkley 1988).

In the past, it was thought that ADHD behaviours were the result of poor disciplinary practices of parents, but most practitioners now believe that negative parenting styles are instead the result of having a child with ADHD in the family (Anastopoulos & Barkley 1992; Hinshaw 2000). This conclusion is supported by the observation that, once the children's behaviour improves—say, in response to medication—the parents' disciplinary style becomes more positive (Wodrich 1994). It also stands to reason that the parents are not the cause in families where one child has the condition and the siblings do not.

The core behaviours occur in a variety of situations but are most noticeable when the children are tired, expected to concentrate for long periods, and are in a group rather than one-to-one situations; when the activity is boring or repetitive; when movement is restricted; and when there is no supervision (Anastopoulos & Barkley 1992).

Gain a comprehensive assessment. Because affected children's behaviour will fluctuate across settings, an accurate diagnosis is possible only when information is gained from many sources, including your own and parents' reports of the children's behaviour, plus developmental and medical assessments. The aims of the latter are to rule out other possible conditions and to gain an understanding of any associated secondary problems, such as language difficulties, learning disabilities and health conditions (Anastopoulos & Barkley 1992).

Medication. For children aged over five years and those with moderate to severe symptoms, medication still appears to have more benefits than any other form of treatment (Anastopoulos & Barkley 1992; Barkley 1988; Fox & Rieder 1993; Goldstein 1995; Hinshaw 2000). Nevertheless, the debate continues about which children benefit most from medication, and at which doses (Levy 1993) while the effects for children aged under five years have not been adequately studied to draw conclusions for this age group.

At higher doses, children are more likely to experience common side effects such as appetite suppression (resulting in slowed growth), nausea, and headaches (Fox & Rieder 1993). Given these potential side-effects, it would seem that, for young childen and those with mild symptoms, drugs should not be the first treatment option. On the other hand, the impact of severe ADHD on affected children and their families might justify administration of drugs. The decision to use medication, then, will depend on (Goldstein & Goldstein 1995):

- the severity of the condition;
- whether other treatments have been tried and have failed;
- the child's age;
- the child's and family's attitude to medication; and
- the ability of parents and caregiver-teachers to supervise a medication regime adequately.

Medication does not have to continue indefinitely: sometimes, children benefit from giving themselves and their family a rest from the symptoms, during which time they can muster their resources to learn how to cope in other ways.

Behavioural guidance. Because children with ADHD lack self-control, the temptation is to try to control their behaviour by using star charts, time out, withdrawal of privileges, and other controlling discipline methods. But you need to remember that these approaches will only teach children to do as they are told—if they worked—whereas these children's problem is that they are not taking charge of their own behaviour. If you manage their behaviour for them, they will never learn how to do it for themselves. Furthermore, research has shown that the use of a guidance approach by parents improves the children's social skilfulness and reduces antisocial and defiant behaviour (Hinshaw 2000).

Therefore, I recommend the methods described in Chapters 7-10 to teach affected children how to take charge of their own behaviour. Approaches should focus particularly on teaching emotional self-control—particularly anger management, adjusting dysfunctional thinking, and self-monitoring (Hinshaw 2000). It might take longer than usual and could be more difficult for these children to learn to think before they act, but in my view the alternative of controlling them externally will never teach them how to.

Also, many children who are diagnosed with ADD or ADHD feel unable to meet the expected standards for their behaviour and so, while improving their skills is important, it is also crucial to ensure that your expectations of the children are appropriate (Zentall 1989).

Assist the children's social difficulties. These children's social difficulties can be their most significant problem. Their peers tend to reject them because of their physical aggression—which is ten times higher than normal—and verbal aggression, which is three times higher (Goldstein 1995). Not surprisingly, this behaviour leads both to difficulties with establishing friendships and, even more importantly, to sustaining friendships—except perhaps with other children who are experiencing similar difficulties (Barkley 1988). See Chapters 5 and 12 for ways to encourage prosocial skills.

Dietary management. The research evidence for dietary restrictions is still scant. Only some children appear to benefit from dietary modifications. However, the lack of uniform effects from changed diets could come about because, although the children's outward symptoms are similar, each child's trigger food might be different. Unless the particular food to which individuals are sensitive is removed from their diet, the symptoms would remain; removing an irrelevant food would obviously produce no improvement. (The categories of suspect foods were outlined in Chapter 11.)

Food intolerances are considered more likely in children who have severe symptoms of the condition and who have family members with allergic conditions such as eczema, asthma or migraines (Goldstein 1995). Another potential dietary trigger is a link between ADD/ADHD and high insulin production. When too much insulin is produced, affected children's blood sugar levels drop too low for adequate brain functioning. In response, blood (containing the fuel, sugar) is directed away from non-essential areas of the brain: namely, away from the pre-frontal lobes (Blum & Mercugliano 1997). The symptoms of ADD/ADHD then surface. This pattern is most likely in children who have a family member with diabetes, who crave carbohydrates, or whose symptoms appear around two hours after the last meal. Blood tests for glucose tolerance and serum insulin levels can flag hyperinsulinemia as a potential cause. Treatment can involve a low-carbohydrate diet, or a diet in which every meal contains at least 50% protein and not more than 50% carbohydrates. Naturally, medical advice is essential before parents implement any dietary restrictions for their children.

Elimination diets or orthodox medical or homeopathic tests can diagnose food intolerances. (Your local Allergy Association or Attention-Deficit Disorders Association will have lists of practitioners who are interested in this field.) Although medical evidence is still uncertain, many practitioners consider that at least some children who have been diagnosed with ADHD can benefit from dietary modifications, and that these children may suffer unnecessarily if we withhold dietary management while awaiting unequivocal evidence.

Support parents. ADHD excites a large share of scepticism and victim blaming. As a result of their child's demanding behaviours and their own reduced confidence about meeting these, parents of children with ADHD often feel stressed and parent in ways that appear to be exacerbating their child's difficulties. Alternatively, some parents report that their child has ADHD-like behaviour at home but you see none of it at the centre, thus making it seem as if the parents are less competent than you. But part of this syndrome is that the children's behaviour fluctuates and is responsive to structure, so differences across settings are inevitable. Also, many children behave less well for their parents in the confidence that their parents will love them anyway. And you can expect that parents will be more stressed by a child's unrelenting difficulties and so are more likely than you are to find these overwhelming.

Therefore, resist the temptation to doubt parents. Exchange information with them about what works and doesn't work for each of you; if they appear to be in need and like to read, suggest some books that might give them some additional disciplinary strategies. Finally, you could ask their permission to speak directly to their child's medical specialists, so that you are better equipped to understand their child's condition and treatment regime.

Children with disabilities

Some disabilities are associated with very challenging behaviour and will need to be dealt with in light of the constraints of the children's condition. For example, children whose disability comprises cardiac conditions or asthma generally cannot be allowed to get emotionally hysterical, as can sometimes happen during tantrums. On the whole, however, children with disabilities will profit from the same behavioural guidance approaches as typically developing children. At the same time, you can have a role in supporting their parents.

I have no data to support this but, in my experience, children with intellectual disabilities (mental retardation, in U.S. terms) tend to be able to behave at a more sophisticated level than their cognitive skills might dictate. In group settings in particular, they can observe how other children are conducting themselves and abide by the same code, whereas independently they might not remember expectations for their behaviour. As depicted in Figure 13.1(a) (see p. 164), then, I have found that the children's behaviour exceeds their intellectual skills but generally does not attain the level of their actual age.

Adjust your program, as required

Children with atypical needs will have many curricular requirements in common with their age mates but also require some adjustments to the environment, the teaching and learning processes you employ, and the content of their program. As this text is not devoted to curricular issues, individualisation of programs will not be detailed here but must be mentioned as a means of avoiding behavioural disruptions that occur when children's needs are not being met.

Consider placement

Placement decisions centre on the age and ability levels of surrounding children. In terms of age, to foster modelling, children with developmental delays might be suited to placement within a group of younger children with similar developmental levels to their own as they are more likely to copy the behaviour of children whom they regard as similar to themselves. On the other hand, typically developing three-year-olds are less able than four-year-olds to adjust their communication style to accommodate older children with delays, in which case younger children might not be ideal social companions (Guralnick et al. 1998).

Even among a group of younger children, there are still likely to be differences not only in *what* the various children can achieve but in *how* they achieve it (McCollum & Bair 1994). Also, if the children with disabilities are physically large, they might look out of place among a group of younger children, which raises questions about whether such a placement is suitable.

On the other hand, placement alongside age mates can put children with delayed development in danger if, for instance, they are still mouthing or eating materials such as glue or nails which are part of the regular children's activities, or if the climbing equipment that suits typical children is dangerous to them. If the children with disabilities are unsteady on their feet, they can be scared of being knocked over by very active children and so lose confidence in moving about independently.

Insist on considerate behaviour

It can be tempting to allow children's disabilities to excuse poor behaviour. But when you expect less of people, you gain less for them. And if you allow them to behave inconsiderately, you will give them a dual disability: the original one and an antisocial habit that will lead to rejection by peers. Moreover, surrounding children have the right not to be victimised by another's behaviour, even when no malice is intended. Therefore it is important to understand the difficulties under which children with disabilities are functioning and to compensate for these with increased support but, wherever possible, not to make undue allowances for them or require surrounding children to tolerate intolerable behaviour.

Give additional opportunities for self-determination

Whereas non-disabled babies see a toy and manage to roll over to inspect it, children with physical difficulties cannot act on that impulse. So, to avoid teaching them that they are helpless, it is absolutely crucial that babies who have physical disabilities receive early physiotherapy treatment. Not only does being able to move teach them about whatever they are exploring, but it teaches them that they can plan to do something and carry it out: they learn that they can learn. Numerous opportunities to exercise choice over those things they can control will also reinforce this disposition to master themselves. This will be influential in their development but also will affect their willingness to exercise control over their emotions and thus their own behaviour.

Make feedback concrete, if necessary

Although throughout this text I have advocated for natural reinforcers and the use of acknowledgment rather than praise, on rare occasions, I have had to contrive some feedback. This has been necessary for those rare children with severe disabilities, particularly in the language domain, for whom verbal feedback is meaningless and so who need some physical evidence that they are achieving the many small steps towards success. In these cases, I have used stars, placing them inside an outline of children's favourite cartoon character—not as a reward for listening to instructions or acting thoughtfully, or whatever—but as a form of *evidence* of that achievement. Placing the sticker on the drawing 'punctuates' the teaching session, as it were, allowing us to pause and highlight the children's efforts. Once the character is filled with stickers, the children have some physical evidence to remind themselves of their achievements. Meanwhile, the feedback is still informative, not judgmental. It comprises such comments as 'Congratulations! You did it!' or 'Wow. Did you know you could listen so carefully?' or 'How did you do that?' or 'I think you can be proud of that . . . Here's another star to remind you that you did it'. This practice might seem similar to delivering rewards but the intent is to help the children recognise their own achievements by giving them visual information when verbal feedback is not meaningful enough to them.

Support the parents

Children's early years are often the time when parents first encounter their child's additional needs. This means that, at this time, parents may be experiencing an array of conflicting emotions. Some parents may grieve about the loss of their fantasised perfect baby; some grieve for the loss of control over their own circumstances because they now have to defer to the decisions of service providers; some grieve about the changes in their own personal circumstances—such as when a mother who was planning to return to paid employment now finds that she cannot do so (Porter & McKenzie 2000); and, most poignant of all, many grieve for the limitations that the disability imposes on their child.

Whatever their initial emotions, over time, most parents adjust to their unanticipated circumstances, particularly when they have support from within and outside their family—and many come to appreciate the positive contributions that their child makes to their lives (Grant et al. 1998; Sandler & Mistretta 1998; Stainton & Besser 1998). But in these early days they may still be experiencing uncertainty, anger, depression or isolation arising from the sense that no one else understands what they are going through. They might lack confidence in their ability to meet their child's additional needs, and experience sheer exhaustion from going the rounds of many professionals in an attempt to achieve a diagnosis and design a suitable intervention.

Mothers in particular can need permission to look after themselves and give themselves time to experience and resolve their emotions. They often busy themselves so much with the daily care of their child that they neglect their own needs, so they might need encouragement to use day care to give them a respite from the extra demands of parenting their child with additional needs. Using alternative care can free them to attend to their marriage, the needs of any other children in the family, and their own requirement to stay in touch with family and friends so that they have a well-balanced life that will equip them to offer their best to their child.

Empower parents

For some parents, their encounter with disability services will be their first experience of having to defer to expert opinion; others may have experienced this in other spheres of their lives and are already demoralised or bitter about helping agencies. Their vulnerability to expert opinion is probably inevitable but you can help by reminding parents that they are the experts about their own child and that only they know their aspirations for their son or daughter. Make sure that you do not aggravate their powerlessness by imposing your views on them and undermining their confidence, and help them to locate professionals who will treat them similarly.

Provide information as requested

When they are ready, give parents any information that they are seeking to help them make decisions about their child's care. When parents seem uncertain about their child's condition, you might gather information by reading or by talking with disability specialists or representatives of parent support groups. At the same time, be careful not to hurry parents into dealing with both present and future problems all at once: parents of non-disabled children do not have to anticipate their adolescents' drug use and unemployment at the same time as learning to parent a new baby, so parents of children with disabilities should not have to cope with everything at once either.

Parents of children with additional needs tend to want information about (Porter & McKenzie 2000: 98):

- their child's additional needs;
- typical and atypical child development;
- how to recognise and respond to any atypical cues that their child uses to communicate with them (Guralnick 1991);
- their child's learning characteristics and future potential or prognosis;
- how to support their child at home;
- how to play with their child at home;
- the range of available services such as therapy services, respite care, relevant community activities, financial assistance to offset additional costs, future schooling options;
- behaviour management strategies;
- managing their emotional reactions and that of other family members; and
- parent support groups.

Keep in mind, however, that many parents will already have learned more about their child's disability and about disability services than you will know, so information exchange should be two-way.

Do not impose a formal teaching role on parents

Parental support for their children's education is crucial to the success of interventions with children with disabilities. However, this can most profitably take the form of joint planning of their child's program, rather than having parents act as formal teachers of their children, as the latter can actually be counter-productive (Ramey & Ramey 1992; White et al. 1992). Parents in formal teaching roles can become distressed to see their child struggling to be successful, can find that the time involved interferes intolerably with their other family responsibilities, or can cause them to focus on being a formal instructor instead of emotionally nurturing their child. Therefore, any educational or behavioural programs that are instituted at your centre must not be imposed on parents at home.

Secure relevant services

Children with disabilities often require a complex array of services, including direct therapy. You can assist here by recommending relevant specialists and, where appropriate, carrying out in your setting the activities they devise. This gives children additional practice of the skills they are struggling to learn and allows them to exercise these in natural settings, which makes it more likely that they will transfer these into community settings as well.

Support siblings

Children whose brother or sister requires their parents' constant attention or who worry about their parents can sometimes take on responsibilities beyond their years for looking after others. This can result in very caring behaviour towards their sibling and others, alternated with careless—even endangering—behaviour. So if children in your care have a sibling with a disability, ensure that their time at your centre provides a respite from any additional responsibilities they might be adopting.

Involve grandparents, as appropriate

Many grandparents were brought up in an era when people with disabilities were hidden away. As a result, they might have very little knowledge—and many misconceptions—about their grandchild's disability. This can cause them to doubt their ability to help look after the child and might cause them to question how the child's parents are handling his or her additional needs. So, with the parents' permission, it can help to invite grandparents to any meetings so that they can update their knowledge and ask their own questions about their grandchild's condition and needs.

Provide extra supports at times of transition

Times of transition—such as from preschool to school—can be a particular challenge as parents might revisit their earlier grief at their child's disability and a renewed despair at the fact that the next placement will not meet his or her needs perfectly (Bentley-Williams & Butterfield 1996; Fowler et al. 1991). Because of their extra vulnerability, they might have developed more than the usual reliance on their caregivers and are reluctant to lose your support. To assist them to move on to the next service, you can plan with them well in advance for a move, and gradually introduce both the child and parents to the new setting—as long as this does not go on for so long that the children seem for prolonged periods not to belong either in the former or the new setting.

Gather supports for yourself

It is often claimed that caregivers' attitudes are the crucial factor in their ability to cater appropriately for children with atypical needs but, in fact, your ability to provide for these children is mostly influenced by the supports that are available to you (MacMullin & Napper 1993). For you to be effective in providing for children's atypical requirements, you will need access to sufficient staff to give children individual attention as required; planning time; training in exceptional needs; advice from specialist personnel such as speech pathologists, psychologists, and physio- and occupational therapists; and for these various services to be coordinated (Buysse et al. 1998; Dinnebeil et al. 1998; McDonnell et al. 1997; Stoiber et al. 1998).

Explain the disability to peers

When parents first enrol their child with additional needs, it will be important to gain their permission to explain to the other children about the child's disability. The other children will need clear, straightforward information about the disability, and will need permission to ask questions about it. At times, it will also be important to comment on how the child with a disability is similar to the other children.

Young children might be scared of 'catching' a disability or assume that it imposes limitations on all aspects of the child's development—for instance, when they see that a child cannot walk, they might think that he or she has intellectual delays as well (Doherty-Derkowski 1995). As a result, they might not consider the child a suitable playmate, or they might be too helpful. To overcome this, convey your confidence that the child with disabilities has many capabilities, as the children will copy your behaviour towards the child, and will be over-solicitous and protective only if you are.

Finally, it is crucial that you do not burden young children with caring for a child who has a disability. Not only would it patronise the child him or herself, but it would be too much responsibility for the other children. One way to avoid this is by showing the children how to talk naturally to a child who has a disability.

Communicate with parents of the non-disabled children

Parents of the non-disabled children in your care have a right to reassurance that a child with a disability will not require a disproportionate amount of staff time, resulting in reduced care of their own child. However, you will need to decide on a case-by-case basis how much information you should tell the other parents about the attendance of a child with a disability, as disclosure could create unnecessary anxiety or be construed as a tacit invitation for protests (Chandler 1994); conversely, if you do not discuss the issue with your parent group, some might feel that you are not receptive to their legitimate concerns. Your decision about disclosure will need to be made with sensitivity to parents whose child has additional needs. But a positive byproduct of communicating with the parent group is that many will now feel comfortable approaching the parent whose child has a disability, thus reducing that parent's isolation.

Gifted children

Giftedness simply means that children are developing at a faster pace than usual—at least one-third faster—such that a three-year-old is as able in one or more developmental domains as the typical four-year-old. It is usually considered that 3%–5% of the population are gifted to this or a greater extent.

Gifted children have a lower than usual incidence of behavioural difficulties (Cornell et al. 1994; Gallucci 1988), particularly when their atypical educational and social-emotional needs are being met. Because they are able to anticipate outcomes at young ages, they tend to be less impulsive and thus less accident-prone than age mates. Nevertheless, some have heightened activity levels that cause them to seek constant stimulation, which can be demanding on their caregivers; some react emotionally to feeling different from their peers; most have emotional development that is in advance of their years but nevertheless not as advanced as their gifted skills; and some become bored easily in a regular program and so find things to do that unintentionally disrupt others (Porter 1999a).

Figure 13.1: Behavioural levels of children with atypical development

(a) **Children with intellectual disabilities**

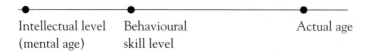

Intellectual level   Behavioural   Actual age
(mental age)   skill level

(b) **Gifted children**

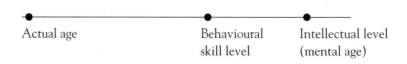

Actual age   Behavioural   Intellectual level
                                       skill level   (mental age)

If no intellectual peers are available to them, these children can appear to be disengaged socially; if the educational program is not challenging for them intellectually, they might flit from one activity to another, never really becoming engrossed in the activities on offer. As a result of this lack of social and active engagement, it can appear that the children have delayed rather than advanced development so careful observation is necessary to recognise the signs of giftedness (such as those listed in Box 13.1).

As a result of being 'out of sync' with their environment and peers, gifted children can display emotional outbursts that appear immature, especially compared with their more mature behaviour at other times. In an attempt to receive stimulation, they can develop deep attachments to their parents, other adults or gifted peers but, at the same time, appear not to develop a breadth of attachments that you might see in less able children. They can be devastated by the absence of a close friend, as they do not find age mates as companionable as intellectual peers.

In turn, these behaviours tend to be misinterpreted as evidence that the children are not gifted or that they are 'not ready' to move up to the next group in the centre or to start school early. However, coupled with the signs of advanced development mentioned in Box 13.1, this pattern of behaviour suggests the need for some program adjustments.

Provide an individualised program, where required. If there are many children in your centre who are very able learners, individuals might not need to be singled out for individualised programming as your centre will be providing for them as a group; if, however, individual children who are bright have few or no age mates at their intellectual level in attendance, you will need to provide an individualised program in order to meet their needs.

Acknowledge, but do not praise. If you praise the advanced achievements of gifted children within others' hearing, the surrounding children might feel discouraged, as they will not be able to attain the same sophisticated performances. Instead, acknowledge the effort involved in producing each child's work, and highlight the dispositions that they are exercising, such as when they are persistent, have planned how to go about a task, have solved problems, negotiated with others, and so on.

Do not emphasise fine hand skills. Although advanced in other domains, gifted children's eye-hand skills are typically nearer the average (Tannenbaum 1983). They also have more ideas than usual for their age, and the discrepancy between what they can imagine and what they can put on paper can be demoralising. Therefore, I suggest that although you must

Box 13.1: Indicators of advanced development in young children

The following characteristics and behaviours can indicate advances in children's development during the early childhood years. However, it must be said that some of these signs can be due to reasons other than giftedness—and that no gifted child will display all of the signs. Furthermore, it is not clear which behaviours are essential to giftedness and which are unnecessary—and we have insufficient knowledge to allow us to give extra weight to the most important features (Perleth et al. 2000).

Nevertheless, the fundamental criterion for defining giftedness is that the children's development (in at least one developmental domain) is proceeding at least one-third faster than expected at that age—such that a three-year-old more closely resembles at least a four-year-old's development.

Cognitive (thinking) skills
Children who are developing significantly ahead of age in their intellectual abilities may show an array of the following behaviours. They:

- achieve developmental milestones early (at least one-third sooner than expected);

(Continued)

Box 13.1: *(Continued)*

- learn quickly;
- observe the environment keenly;
- are active in eliciting stimulation from the environment—sometimes leading to reliance on parents to act as 'input' for them;
- may read, write or use numbers in advanced ways (although this is not all that common: if the children are reading during the preschool years, they are likely to be highly gifted, if they are not reading early, that may not be significant);
- show advanced preferences for books and films, unless too sensitive to older themes;
- have quick and accurate recall. (Although this is necessary, having a good memory is not sufficient on its own to lead to giftedness);
- can recall skills and information introduced some time ago;
- possess deeper knowledge than other children: they have information on more topics, and know more about those topics;
- have an ability to teach other children (although they might become irritated if others appear not to learning, and may have difficulty describing the steps involved in tasks as they themselves did not need to learn them in a stepwise fashion but were competent almost immediately);
- understand abstract concepts (for example, death or time) early;
- are imaginative or creative (not just with artistic pursuits but in their problem-solving as well); and
- have an advanced sense of humour (because they understand incongruity, which is the basis of humour).

Learning style
As well as *what* they are able to achieve, young children who are learning at a faster pace than usual typically go about tasks in sophisticated ways—that is, *how* they achieve is exceptional. They:

- are motivated, curious, and seek to understand;
- will focus intensely on an area of interest, as long as there is sufficient challenge;
- have wide-ranging interests;
- are alert (sometimes resulting in poor sleeping patterns and sometimes in sound sleep as a result of expending their energy all day);

(Continued)

Box 13.1: *(Continued)*

- respond to novel stimuli and get used quickly to repetitive activities;
- have a longer than usual concentration span on challenging topics of interest (but may 'flit' from one activity to another if activities are not challenging enough);
- use metacognitive skills early to manage their own thinking processes;
- have a clear understanding of cause-and-effect;
- possess good planning skills;
- have an internal locus of control;
- are less impulsive than usual for their age (and so have fewer injuries than usual);
- can be independent when working at challenging, non-routine tasks but highly dependent when bored; and
- can think logically.

Speech and language skills

Children whose advances fall within the verbal domain tend to show the following characteristics. They:
- comprehend language early;
- use advanced speech—in terms of vocabulary, grammar and clear articulation;
- will use metaphors and analogies (for example, when hanging upside-down on a jungle gym will announce that they are a bat);
- will make up songs or stories spontaneously;
- can modify their language to suit less mature children;
- use language for a real exchange of ideas and information at an early age; and
- can carry out instructions to do several things in succession.

Motor abilities

Children with advanced physical skills may display the following characteristics. They:
- display early development of motor skills, particularly those that are under cognitive control (such as balance)—in contrast with those (such as stamina) which are purely physical;
- can locate themselves within the environment;

(Continued)

Box 13.1: *(Continued)*

- have an early awareness that there is a left and right, without necessarily being able to name these accurately;
- may have average fine motor skills, which means that these lag behind their other developmental skills, leading to some children's reluctance to draw or write and later to untidy handwriting through a lack of practice and reduced motivation;
- can put together new or difficult puzzles (particularly if visually advanced, in contrast with children who prefer to learn auditorally);
- can take apart and reassemble objects with unusual skill;
- can make interesting shapes or patterns with objects; and
- have high levels of physical energy (sometimes leading to queries about motoric or vocal ADHD).

Social skills

Some gifted children are particularly adept at relationships and are tuned in to other people and their feelings. These children often:

- have highly developed empathy for others;
- are less egocentric than usual—that is, can interpret accurately what is bothering others;
- have advanced play interests;
- can play games with rules earlier than usual;
- may form close, reciprocal friendships from a young age (as long as intellectual peers are available);
- seek out older children or adults for companionship if intellectual peers are not available;
- might withdraw to solitary play if intellectual peers are not available;
- are often sought out by other children—that is, others feel drawn to them but nevertheless the gifted children themselves might not feel as warmly disposed to others who are not 'soul mates';
- can display leadership skills, although in their early years they might not have the maturity to exercise tact with those whom they are leading;
- develop moral reasoning and judgment early (although might not act accordingly unless circumstances facilitate that); and

(Continued)

Box 13.1: *(Continued)*

- take an early interest in social issues involving injustices (sometimes leading to the need for media blackouts in times of wars and other world crises).

Emotional and behavioural characteristics

Finally, some children whose development is advanced have been described as showing the following emotional features. They:

- can be emotionally sensitive, intense and responsive. (As this can be a response to frustration at their uneven developmental levels across a range of skill domains, any children with atypical development may be similarly emotional.);
- develop fears early;
- develop their self-concept early and so are aware from a young age of being different from others (from perhaps as young as two years old);
- are self-confident in their strong domains but less confident in their less advanced domains;
- might be perfectionist, in the sense of seeking to achieve at high levels;
- can be over-sensitive to criticism;
- may become frustrated at their lesser skills, which can lead to emotional or behavioural outbursts;
- may accept responsibility usually given only to older children (which is important not to exploit, as the children may not be free to develop fully while taking care of others' business); and
- are non-conformist—and so do not take kindly to authoritarian forms of discipline whereby they are expected to do as they are told without an explanation.

SOURCE: ADAPTED FROM PORTER (1999A: 74-76)

encourage drawing and other fine hand skills, you should not demand that gifted children concentrate on these or use fine hand proficiency as a requirement for advancement to the next level of education.

Tell gifted children the truth. Children whose development is significantly advanced can become aware very early in life that they are different from other children (Clark 1997; Harrison 1999). Therefore, you will need to explain to gifted children that they feel different because some things about them are different. Avoiding the label 'gifted' because of its emotiveness, you can simply explain that their brains can learn more quickly than other children's. Without putting them down, explain that this does not make them better than anyone else—just different.

Explain the frustration of uneven development. Some children become frustrated that they are not equally good at everything. As already mentioned, for instance, most children with advanced development nevertheless have average fine motor skills and so their drawing and handwriting is not advanced. I explain this to them by saying that, while brains can grow up at various speeds, hands can grow up only at body speed and so sometimes, although the children have an idea of what they want to do, their hands are not yet grown up enough to be able to do it. So they will need to be patient with themselves while their hands grow up.

Expect some dependence. Young gifted children can become dependent on adults for stimulation and to help them with self-care tasks such as dressing, especially after they know how to do the activity and it holds no new intellectual challenge for them. Their resulting dependence can be frustrating and can result in separation difficulties, as they are reluctant to leave the parent who has translated their needs to the outside world and interpreted the outside world to them. To deal with these issues, continue to expect age-appropriate independence, but give more support when needed. As for the separation difficulties, see Chapter 11 for its suggestions.

Understand perfectionism. Perfectionism is the engine that drives gifted children to achieve to high standards, and so it is not dysfunctional for them—except when outsiders grow frustrated with it or when the children themselves become dissatisfied with achievements that are excellent but imperfect (Parker & Adkins 1995). The solution is not to try to placate children when they feel disappointed in their performances but to reflect what they are feeling. Next, you might give your opinion that what they have done is of high quality but suggest that if they feel it needs to be improved, then perhaps they could have another try—either immediately or after taking a break from it. In other words, the goal is not to get them to lower their standards, but to help them meet their goals.

Teach children about boredom. With most children, we try not to make tasks too difficult but, with gifted children, it is equally important that we do not expect too little of them and make tasks too easy, such that they become bored. Having said that, once expectations are realistic, it can be necessary to teach children that boredom is of their own making and that, if they feel 'bored', only they can solve that by choosing to engage enthusiastically in something worthwhile. It is also important to emphasise that, like everyone else, gifted children need time to consolidate and practise the skills they already have, so do not need to be learning new things all the time.

Help them avoid loneliness. It can be hard to find friends for young gifted children because they often need to play with older children, most of whom already attend preschool or school. For this reason, it can be useful to link young children up with other gifted children of their age. Not only will this help them to be less isolated and lonely, but it will give parents access to a support group. (See also the suggestions in Chapter 12 for isolated children.)

Explain other children's behaviour. Many gifted children develop a sense of justice before others of their age. They understand how to share, take turns, or use words to solve problems long before their age mates. As a result, they assume that another child's aggression, lack of empathy, or lack of planning are a deliberate attempt to hurt them instead of the normal developmental ignorance that it is—and so they are more deeply hurt than average learners would be. Therefore, explain that other children are still making mistakes because they cannot learn as quickly as the gifted children can, but that others do not mean to hurt them by these errors.

Consider early entry. Fifty years of international research confirms that if young gifted children are lonely because in their present setting they cannot locate friends at their intellectual level, and are intellectually frustrated because they cannot receive the educational stimulation they require, they are better placed early amongst children who are older than themselves (Porter 1999a). This is usually called 'acceleration' but is really only a case of providing a placement that is developmentally appropriate (Feldhusen 1989). When considering early entry to a new setting, each child's academic, social and emotional readiness needs to be weighed up individually, which is too detailed to outline here (see instead Porter 1999a). But worries about the effects of early exit should not determine decisions about early entry: we cannot hold children back now on the off-chance that problems might occur later.

Develop realistic expectations for gifted children. It can be difficult to know what to expect of gifted children as their mature behaviour can deceive adults into expecting that of them all the time. Those with advanced language can be deceptive in that they understand adult ideas intellectually while not being ready emotionally to cope.

To overcome this, remind yourself repeatedly of the children's actual age, and realise that their emotional status is likely to fall somewhere between their actual age and their developmental level: it will not quite keep up with their advanced intellect (see Figure 13.1b). And if you do expect a lot of them for their age, compensate for this by increasing the amount of support you give them.

Encourage them to give themselves permission to shine. Once they understand that they feel different because they actually are different, you can encourage them to 'give themselves permission to shine' (this line having been borrowed from a current popular song). The children can be tactful and not parade their skills in front of others—without, on the other hand, hiding their light under a bushel to protect others from their advanced abilities.

Establish clear boundaries between adult and child business. Children with advanced awareness might begin to involve themselves in adult issues. You might be able to advise parents how to guard against this—such as by limiting exposure to news bulletins; ensuring that adults do not discuss unresolved family issues in the children's hearing; and giving children permission to act their age in most things, even when some of their development is advanced of this.

Conclusion

When children have known disabilities—say, a vision impairment—we would not instruct them to overcome their difficulties by demanding: 'Use your eyes!'. Even when children have less obvious difficulties, instead of blaming them for their behaviours, we need to help them to circumvent the obstacles under which they are functioning. This does not translate into making undue allowances for them but to understanding that they are struggling and increasing the support that we give them so that they can make the best use of their residual skills.

When children's development is not typical, it is crucial to get some professional advice early in their lives. This avoids one problem spreading to other areas of their life—such as when their inability to speak or understand language causes social difficulties for them. It also avoids having to undo some of their dysfunctional patterns—such as when children with physical disabilities learn to slide around on their bottoms and then become frustrated when first learning to walk and finding it a much slower way of getting around.

So, if you are concerned that individual children's behaviour or development seems atypical, ask their parents for permission to refer the children to a specialist. The earlier an intervention is initiated, the more effective it can be.

Suggested further reading

For information on catering for children with either disabilities or advanced development:

Porter, L. (Ed.) (2002a). *Educating young children with additional needs*. Sydney: Allen and Unwin.

Porter, L. (Ed.) (2002b). *Educating young children with special needs*. London: Paul Chapman/Thousand Oaks, CA: SAGE.

For a theoretical and practical overview of special education for young children:

Allen, K.E. & Schwartz, I.S. (2001). *The exceptional child: Inclusion in early childhood education*. (4th ed.) Albany, NY: Delmar.

For practical recommendations for catering for children with disabilities:

Sandall, S.R. & Schwartz, I.S. (2002). *Building blocks for teaching preschoolers with special needs*. Baltimore, MD: Paul H. Brookes.

For a detailed discussion of the needs of gifted children:

Porter, L. (1999). *Gifted young children: A guide for teachers and parents*. Sydney: Allen and Unwin/Buckingham, UK: Open University Press.

For a clear overview of ADHD written for lay or professional audiences:

Green, C. & Chee, K. (1997). *Understanding ADHD: A parent's guide to attention-deficit hyperactivity disorder in children*. Sydney: Random House.

14

●●●

Family issues

Children cannot and should not be protected from all stressful situations; however, exposure to such situations must fit [their] ability to deal with stressful circumstances.

GOWEN & NEBRIG (2002: 32)

This chapter suggests how you can guide children when their disruptive behaviour appears to stem from family malfunctioning. Although some of these challenges—such as parental separation or child abuse—might seem to be modern phenomena, today's families actually differ very little from those in the past (Waters & Crook 1993): it is simply that we are now talking more than we once did about some of the problems they experience. As a result, there are fewer secrets, which means that children no longer suffer the burden of not being able to disclose what is happening in their lives. And once we know what conditions the children are experiencing, we can make an extra effort to offer a steady emotional base when one is not presently available to them at home, and thus minimise their long-term distress.

General guidelines for supporting stressed children

You have a dual role when assisting children whose families are functioning in stressful circumstances: the prime one being to assist and advocate for the children, and a less direct role of supporting their parents.

Understand but do not excuse antisocial behaviour

While understanding that certain children's disruptive behaviour is being provoked by difficult living conditions, you nevertheless cannot allow these circumstances to excuse antisocial behaviour. If the children are allowed to develop antisocial habits, they will then be doubly disadvantaged. So, increase the amount of support you offer troubled children so that they can meet your behavioural expectations, rather than lowering your demands.

Guide the children's behaviours

Use non-punitive means for correcting behaviours that are being provoked by stress. Children living in stressed families are already suffering adverse circumstances and, sometimes, punitive forms of discipline, so need to experience a positive alternative. As we cannot always detect which children are being disadvantaged by their home circumstances, it is safer to use a guidance approach with them all.

Build warm relationships with troubled children

Children who are displaying troublesome behaviour almost appear to invite rejection from all those around them. Do not allow their behaviour to alienate you, however, as that will compound their difficulties. Instead, work extra diligently to build a warm relationship with the children, whereby you respect their experience of the world and the things that interest them. The children might not immediately warm to you and thus improve their behaviour—so you will have to persist longer than they think you will.

Be a resiliency mentor

Resilience does not come about by avoiding adversity but by receiving the necessary supports to overcome it in a way that enhances children's self confidence and faith in their own ability to master challenges (Rutter 1985). You can boost their confidence by expressing faith that they will be able to overcome their present difficulties and teaching them how to overcome adversity by using the problem-solving skills that they already possess but perhaps under-utilise (Ryan 1989).

Assist distressed children to separate appropriately

Children with disturbed attachment to their parents—perhaps as a result of abuse or neglect—often have mixed emotions at separation from their parents (Gowen & Nebrig 2002). They will need extra advance preparation to separate and the parents may need some guidance about how to rebond emotionally with their child upon reunion. While these children are in your care, to compensate for neglectful parents' lack of responsiveness, you will need to be highly responsive in your caregiving so that the children learn that they can ask for and receive care when they need it.

Help children to grow down

When their families are stressed by either short-term crises or longer-term disadvantaging living conditions, children are often given, or sometimes take on for themselves, the responsibility of looking after their parents. This is too much responsibility for such young people and, as a result, they might display very mature behaviour at times but then, like a kettle that has been simmering and then suddenly boils over, they display unexpected outbursts. They are having to act too maturely for their years—and the strain eventually overwhelms them.

If individual children in your care seem to be displaying signs of bearing too much responsibility for their parents' welfare, you could assess this by asking the children about who is responsible for whom in the family. The well-adjusted situation is where they can report that Mum looks after herself, her partner (where relevant) and the children; Dad looks after himself, his partner and the children; while the children look after their teddy or dolls and help look after the family pets. If instead the children answer that they look after one or both of their parents, you might tactfully draw this to their parents' attention. Many times the parents do not realise that their children are worried about them and, once aware that this is the case, can reassure the children that there is no need for concern: the parents are in command of the situation, even if it is difficult and even if they do not yet know how they will proceed. The parents could thank the children for their concern but remind them that they need all their energy to grow up in the many ways that children develop, and so must devote themselves to that rather than to worrying about adult affairs.

Meanwhile, there might be an opportunity to remind parents that whatever their emotional or financial concerns, these are not their children's business and so they must resist discussing these with their children. Because they *are* children, they do not have the skills to be their parent's friend. Also, encourage the parents to look after themselves (for example, with special outings or by resting when tired) so that the children have evidence that their parents do not need their protection.

Support stressed parents

Although many aspects of family life will be outside of your control, you can direct parents to community and other agencies that can help them to improve their circumstances. In turn, their child will benefit.

Children who have been bereaved

There is a wide-spread misconception that young children do not feel grief and so do not need assistance when they are bereaved by the death of a family member or close friend. However, erratic, sad or withdrawn behaviour can be observed in reaction to loss—even in babies. This means that you will need an understanding of the grieving process so that, although you cannot relieve children's pain at bereavement, in collaboration with their parents, you can assist them to resolve their emotions.

Expect children to react

We expect someone who has been injured to take some time to get well again, but we sometimes forget that emotional pain needs a recovery period too. In the grieving process, adults go through many emotions over many months, beginning with *shock* and numbness; *depression* and loneliness; *panic* about whether we are going crazy; *anger* at ourselves, at the person we have lost, and at anyone who may have contributed to that loss; *guilt* for what we did or did not do that might have contributed to the loss; and at last, gradual *hope* that we can find a new way to be happy—even if we do not yet know exactly how.

Along the way we might get physical symptoms of our distress and we can have unsettling emotional outbursts. Finally, once we have grown through these normal reactions to grief, we can remember the person we have lost without the searing pain that memory used to bring. We might be left with a new insecurity about the possibility of losing someone again but, at the same time, we also know that we can survive to love again.

Children follow a similar pattern, with some additional elements arising from their immature understandings. Under two-year-olds might feel confused at the dead person's sudden absence or at their parents' distraction with their own grief, and might wander off; preschoolers will not realise that death is permanent and so can seem to be callously ignoring their bereavement but then later can become bewildered as they gradually realise that the deceased person is not going to return; children in the five to eight year age group who have said in anger 'I wish you were dead', are likely to think that they caused the other person's death and might try to be especially good to bring the person back to life; while children over nine years of age will experience the same adult-like reactions as already described, and will be interested in the spiritual aspects of death. Finally, adolescents are likely to want to talk about their loss with their peers, but they still need their parents to be available to them as well. Adolescents might worry that someone else in the family could die or leave, which is a particular concern if their parents' marriage is unhappy at the time.

Talk openly about death with children

When young children in your care have been bereaved, it is almost inevitable that in the natural course of events they will talk with you about it, or you might bring the subject up if you feel that the children seem not to be coping. In either case, you will need to talk with their parents about what they would like you to say to the children.

The children will need very concrete facts about death. For example, many are not aware that death is irreversible and that dead people no longer feel, think or sense. It can be crucial to explain these facts to them as otherwise they can become distressed at the burial or cremation. They might need facts and honest answers to their questions about the circumstances and cause of the death; otherwise they will fill in missing details with their imagination, which can be even more frightening than reality. At a time when parents are too distressed to supply this information to the children, you can help by discussing the circumstances with them yourself. In having these conversations, it is important to keep in mind that children cannot cope with a lot of facts at once but instead need to be 'drip fed' small amounts of information often.

At the time of a bereavement, it can pay to restrict conversations to the physical facts of the person's death, as new spiritual information (even when it is consistent with that being provided by the parents) can be too overwhelming to take in at the time of a bereavement. If the children ask where the person goes, it might be best to suggest that they ask their parents (so that this information is in line with their religious views), but you can comment that the spirit of the deceased person, or the love that they felt for that person lives on in their heart and memories, which will always be there.

Explain that the deceased person did not choose to leave them

Tell children that the person whom they loved died because his body grew very old or he became very *very* sick from an illness or an accident—so sick that nothing could be done to make him better. In the case of the death through illness of a baby or child, you might say that the baby's body hadn't been made properly and so she couldn't live in that body any more. It is important to emphasise that the dead person did not *want* to leave them but that he or she couldn't stay in their body any more.

Recommend that children be involved in the rituals surrounding death

Children need their parents at the time of a death and funeral service, even though their parents are upset. It is more frightening for children to be away from their parents than to attend the funeral and, if kept away, they might assume that they are to blame for the person's death and are being punished for it. Therefore, advise parents to include their children where possible. If the time is past, parents could instead involve children in a memorial to the person they have lost, such as by planting and tending a tree in his or her memory.

Children living in poverty

Children are the most likely of any age group to be living in poverty (with the elderly being the next most probable). In Australia, approximately 20% of children experience poverty (with this figure being higher among Aboriginal children) (Gilding 1997); in the U.S. the rate is 20-30%, depending on how it is calculated (Aber & Ellwood 2001). In terms of relative poverty this U.S. figure is equal highest in the industrialised world (along with Russia); in terms of absolute levels, it is at the median among industrialised nations (Aber & Ellwood 2001).

Poverty has a significant direct effect on young children as that is the time when individuals are most prone to the detrimental developmental effects of inadequate nutrition and stimulation (Bradbury et al. 2001). Sameroff (1990) for instance, reports that the rate of mild intellectual disability (or mental retardation, in US terms) is eight times higher in the U.S. than in Sweden, which he attributes to the superior levels of support available to impoverished families in Sweden.

Furthermore, functioning under the burden of chronic poverty is linked with other risk factors that are detrimental to children—such as poor housing; limited social supports when one lives in a neighbourhood where others are equally stressed; inadequate health care; and low quality child care and educational services (Schaffer 1998). In response, parents might neglect their children's needs as they become caught up in their own issues of survival; inadequate guidance can lead children to develop undesirable peer relationships (selecting friends who are similarly stressed or behaving in antisocial ways) (Schaffer 1998); the parents themselves might develop mental illnesses in response to their trying circumstances; and the parents' relationship can be strained.

The most significant thing that you can do to assist children who are suffering the detrimental effects of poverty is to assist their families to gain the resources they need to fulfil their parenting role adequately (Schaffer 1998). However, they might need considerable encouragement to access such help as many experience official intervention as judgmental, threatening, undermining and authoritarian (Gilding 1997). Meanwhile, for the children themselves, you will need to offer the same types of support as you would for any stressed children, as outlined earlier in this chapter.

Parental separation or divorce

The separation of their parents presents children with many challenges to add to the normal demands of growing up. Over time, they must acknowledge the reality of their parents' separation; disengage from their parents' conflict so that they can get on with their own lives; resolve their grief, anger and any self-blame about the divorce; accept that their parents' separation is permanent; and form realistic expectations for their own future adult relationships (King 1992).

The positive side of this picture is that, now that divorce is possible, parents who are in conflict are able to separate. All the research tells us that children are better off in a divorced family than when living in a family where there is ongoing conflict (Burns & Goodnow 1985). The negative effects on children that we think are caused by divorce instead mainly occur if the conflict between the parents continues after their separation and if the separation exacerbates the family's poverty.

Seek parents' guidance

As is the case with grief over a death, if the parents themselves are too upset to convey information with equanimity, they may be glad for you to supplement the information they can give their children. So ask them what they would like you to say to their child about their separation.

You can emphasise to children who are reacting to a recent parental separation that the parents have left each other—but have not left them. It is the marital relationship—not the parent-child relationship—that is being severed. The children need to know that both parents still love them. Where relevant, they might also need to know whether they will be keeping in touch with both sets of grandparents.

Assist parents in their efforts to support their children

If parents seek your advice, they might find it helpful to receive the following suggestions.

- They should resist belittling their former partner. Even if they feel intense bitterness, they should not talk negatively about their children's absent parent. Family roots are a source of self-esteem for children, so they will devalue themselves if they think that one of their parents is unworthy. Parents might need to recognise that criticising the other parent forces their children to choose between the two of them, with the result that the children will distance themselves from both.
- Even though the parents are no longer living together, they will need to be able to continue to act together in their children's interests so will need to plan their ongoing joint parenting. If they are struggling with this aspect of their separation, they might be open to your recommendation of a counsellor whom they could consult.
- Even if the separation was not of one parent's choosing, that spouse will still have to get on with his or her life. If the parent does not make an effort to design new ways to be happy, the children will worry about their parent and will not be able to get on with their own lives either.
- Recommend that parents avoid additional losses where possible. After the initial upheaval of parental separation, family members can experience additional losses that compound their grief. The children might have to move house or neighbourhoods, or might have to change child care arrangements as their mother increases her work force participation. Sometimes, for financial reasons, the parents cannot avoid these alterations but you might suggest that they space the changes a few months apart if possible, to give the children time to adjust to each new change before another one happens.
- Recommend that the parents be honest when children are genuinely being neglected by their non-custodial parent. It will be useless and hurtful for adults to try to convince children that this is not happening. The custodial parent might sympathise that the absent parent loves them but is 'lazy' about showing his love or, for older children, is 'irresponsible about relationships'. Unfortunately, adults cannot protect children in cases where this is reality, and children only benefit from being allowed to grieve over their very real loss.

Assist children not to become involved in adult issues

When a child's father has died, works away from home for extended periods or has left the family, sometimes well-meaning relatives try to comfort them with the instruction to 'Look after Mum now that Dad is away' or they console a son with the notion that he is 'The man of the house now'. Even without such prompts, some children voluntarily take on the job of looking after their remaining parent. Suggestions for dealing with this issue were given at the beginning of this chapter.

Expect a resurgence of emotions

When children return from access visits with their absent parent, when a parent resumes away-from-home work, or when their custodial parent embarks on a new relationship, you might see many of the same behaviours that were typical of the children during their early grief stages. As you did at the time of their immediate loss, increase the emotional support that you provide, talk with the children about their feelings and, during outbursts, allow them ample time to regain command of their emotions.

Children experiencing family violence

Spouse abuse takes many forms and affects at least one in five families across all social classes, not being confined only to obviously dysfunctioning families (Gilding 1997). *Verbal* abuse is the glue that holds all the other forms in place, and includes putting a spouse down or yelling, while *physical* abuse involves inflicting injury. More subtle forms of abuse include restricting spouses' income or allocation for household expenses (*economic* abuse), restricting their social contacts (*social* abuse), and *sexual* abuse which involves degrading sexual comments, demanding sex and punishing refusals, or causing physical injury during sex.

Just as battered spouses bear the devastating physical and emotional scars of abuse, so too their children suffer from an atmosphere of violence and tension. Furthermore, in homes where spouses are being abused, children are also likely to be recipients of violence (Cummings 1998). The following effects and signs might be observed when children are living with spousal abuse.

- The children might show disrespect for their abused parent, in imitation of their violent parent.
- Their behaviour might then become uncontrollable, as they think that the parent who is being abused does not have enough status to discipline them. They might similarly be dismissive of all other caregivers and so refuse to be guided by you either.

- With so much exposure to power-based conflict, the children often become very bossy or competitive with siblings or peers. They might be aggressive when attempting to solve disputes, either because that is all they have been shown or in reaction to the tension they experience within the home (Cummings 1998).
- They can take on responsibility for protecting the abused parent.

Boys and girls might react differently to domestic violence. Young boys sometimes believe that they have to be aggressive but they worry that someone will find out that they are actually very sensitive instead. They might constantly crave attention. Girls, on the other hand, commonly react to family violence with distrust and fear. They learn to dislike men and marriage. They associate sex with rape and often have strong feelings of aversion about sex in adult life. They can also learn that females have little worth and are helpless to discourage mistreatment.

The children's resulting behavioural difficulties at home can reduce the abused parent's already-low confidence and so he or she does not discipline convincingly; the children might be neglected during the actual violent episode or while the injured parent receives treatment or nurses his or her emotional pain; and, meanwhile, the parents' relationship problems get in the way of finding a joint resolution to the discipline issues with the children.

Assist parents to focus on their children's needs

In amongst their own pain, recipients of violence can understandably lose sight of the fact that the children are seeing and being scared by the violence between their parents. To help them focus on the effects of the violence on the children, when a parent is recounting a violent incident, for example, you could ask questions such as, 'And where was Katy while that (the abuse) was happening? . . . How did she react? . . . How were you able to look after her while feeling so under threat yourself?', and so on (Gowen & Nebrig 2002).

Support abused partners to leave

Violence is such a serious threat to relationships that the spouses will not be able to solve it while one is under threat of more abuse. So recipients of violence will have to leave. But the verbal abuse undermines their confidence that they can live alone. Years of insults convince them that they are helpless—or hopeless. If the parents are looking to you for guidance or support you can assist them to leave by:

- helping them to recognise that they must be very strong to have survived the abuse and to have kept their family functioning;
- asking them in which direction they want to channel this immense strength: into withstanding the violence, or into becoming happy—even if that means leaving?;
- reminding them that their children are suffering in this violent relationship. Love for their children might motivate them to look after themselves as well as the children by leaving (Gowen & Nebrig 2002);
- advising them that most children in abusive families are relieved—not grief-stricken—when their parents separate, especially when that ends the violence; and
- giving them contact details of shelters and counselling agencies that can support them.

Children who are being abused

Child maltreatment takes a number of forms: neglect of children's physical or emotional needs and physical, emotional and sexual abuse. Of these types, neglect constitutes more reported cases than the other forms of maltreatment combined, although many children suffer from multiple forms of abuse simultaneously. This fact complicates calculation of the rate of child abuse, with conservative estimates suggesting that approximately 4% of children are abused (Gilding 1997; Rossman & Rosenberg 1998), while some suggest that the true figure may be up to five times higher, given that so much abuse and neglect goes unreported.

Families who are isolated and lacking in support are more prone to child abuse, while parents' substance abuse is an increasing cause of the neglect of children. Although the use of illicit drugs occurs across all sectors of the community, it is likely to have most impact on those families who are already economically disadvantaged (Hanson & Carta 1995).

The effects of child abuse differ depending on its severity, chronicity, the child's age when it occurs, the relationship between the child and the perpetrator, and the fact that in most cases many types of abuse are co-occurring. When the parents are the perpetrators, the effects of abuse are compounded by the fact that the abuse is happening within dysfunctioning family relationships that are characterised by neglect, indifference, violence, humiliation and terrorisation of children, isolation, corruption of children (as they are enticed into antisocial behaviours), and unreliable parenting (Harter 1998).

A family context where the parents are the perpetrators of abuse or neglect leads to insecure attachments between children and their parents, as the children must continue to rely on their parents for survival at the same time as being under threat from them (Cole-Detke & Kobak 1998; Harter 1998). In this respect, neglected children might be most disadvantaged in that they are less likely to learn how to form attachments to others (Bonner et al. 1992); alternatively, while abused children develop attachments, these are often damaging to them (Steele 1986). Thus, abuse produces developmental and social-emotional impairments and physical injury, with children under the age of five years being at more serious risk of injury than older children (Bonner et al. 1992).

All forms of abuse—physical, emotional and sexual—do not allow children to learn to trust others in their lives, particularly when the perpetrator is a parent. This can have serious emotional effects at the time and in later intimate adult relationships. In terms of their self-esteem, child abuse causes children to see themselves in negative terms and to try to be perfect in an attempt to halt the abuse (Harter 1998). Thus, in the terms discussed in Chapter 4, the children develop a devalued self-concept and unattainably high ideals for themselves.

Some signs of child abuse are listed in Box 14.1. The result of the listed behaviours is that abused children tend to be rejected further by parents or other caregivers. Alternatively, many are ignored in care and preschool settings—unless behaving disruptively, when their interactions with caregivers often comprise disciplinary measures (Hoffman-Plotkin & Twentyman 1984). This emotional neglect compounds the problems these children experience at home and leads to worsening social difficulties throughout childhood (Cole-Detke & Kobak 1998; George & Main 1979; Trickett 1998).

Box 14.1: Signs of child abuse

Emotional signs

- Children who are abused by their parents and who thus develop a dysfunctional attachment to them are often described as highly dependent.
- They tend to know little about their own feelings and do not learn naturally to regulate their anger and aggression—which probably arises from copying their parents' lack of inhibition.
- They display few emotional coping strategies.
- They can display signs of depression or anxiety.

(Continued)

Box 14.1: *(Continued)*

Social signs

- Disturbed attachment to parents can cause neglected or abused children to withdraw from the friendly overtures of caring adults or peers, as their negative experience of relationships teaches them to avoid these.
- Some assault or threaten adults, as they have learned that adults can be dangerous.
- The children learn not to expect nurturance from others so may not approach caregivers for comfort when distressed.
- Many display hostility to others.
- Many lack empathy for others, sometimes even delighting in another child's distress.
- They have limited interactions with peers.
- They are often socially unskilled with peers.
- They exercise few social problem-solving strategies.

Behaviours

If the abuse has been occurring for some time, the behavioural signs are hard to detect, as they too will have been going on for some time. But if the abuse has just begun, you might see a sudden change in abused children's behaviour corresponding with the onset of the abuse.

- When children are abused, their behaviour can regress whereby they display some demanding patterns that were typical of them some time ago, or they adopt new behaviours not seen before.
- Their behaviour is often impulsive as a result of not having learned to regulate their emotions.
- They are frequently disruptive and aggressive.
- Sexually abused children sometimes start being secretive, or talk about a friend or toy who has a secret or to whom something bad is happening. They might ask questions about secrets, and about whether they should tell a secret even when they have promised not to.
- They might display sexualised behaviour such as blatant flirting, excessive touching of their genitals, or perpetrating sexual abuse on surrounding children.

(Continued)

Box 14.1: *(Continued)*

- They might re-enact what is happening to them with their dolls, drawings, or toys or by playing in a sexualised way with other children.
- They might be reluctant to accompany a particular adult.

Physical signs

- Children might have burns, welts, bruises, or fractures whose causes seem inexplicable or are explained unconvincingly.
- Physically abused children might show little response to pain.
- Sexually abused children can have injuries or infections to the genital or anal areas or throat.

Developmental signs

- Abused children often evidence declining development or regression to less mature behaviours, such as when they revert to baby talk, bedwetting or being fearful.
- The children tend not to believe themselves capable of solving problems so they do not apply themselves to these and thus their development is impaired.
- Sexually abused children often display knowledge of adult sexual behaviour that is in advance of their years or developmental level.

SOURCES: HOFFMAN-PLOTKIN & TWENTYMAN 1984; GEORGE & MAIN 1979; GOWEN & NEBRIG 2002; KLIMES-DOUGAN & KISTNER 1990; TRICKETT 1998.

Look for signs of abuse

The above litany of serious effects of abuse makes it essential to report any signs that children might be being abused. To be able to do this, you need to be open to the fact that abuse happens across all social classes: hence the saying:

I wouldn't have seen it, if I hadn't believed it.

Believe children's disclosures of abuse

The single most important thing that you can do to help children when they tell you about being abused, is to believe them. Almost all reports of sexual abuse in particular turn out to be true. This is logical: while children might tell lies to get out of trouble, they seldom tell lies that get themselves into trouble!

Where you see children with unusual injuries, ask them how these happened, and reassure them that help is available. Do not believe ridiculous explanations such as that they have numerous cigarette burns from walking into an adult's cigarette. As they might have been told not to tell anyone about the abuse, reassure them that it is wrong for anyone to tell them to keep a secret forever, and that they can talk to you about anything. Encourage them to talk, but do not force them to confide in you. Do not ask for detailed descriptions of events: experienced investigators are best suited to finding out this information in a way that will not add to the children's distress.

Report child abuse

In only a few cases will children tell you directly that they are being abused (Briggs 1993). Mostly, they will reveal the abuse by accident, or their unusual behaviour will raise your suspicions (Briggs 1993). However the alarm is raised, do not promise to keep the abuse a secret or suggest that the children should forget about what has happened. Their trust has been violated, and they will need to talk about this. Also, ignoring the abuse increases the chances that it will occur again—both to this child and to others in the perpetrator's life. Briggs and McVeity (2000: 29) report that, on average, molesters perpetrate sexual abuse approximately 560 times before being prosecuted!

So, instead of ignoring the abuse or attempting to deal with it yourself, you must notify your local child welfare agency. In so doing, you are not accusing anyone but are simply asking for experts to investigate whether the child is safe. This investigation cannot wait until you have gathered all the necessary evidence. Instead it will be the welfare agency's job to investigate your concerns, which they will aim to do without further victimising the child or those wrongly suspected of being perpetrators.

Be emotionally supportive

You will need to support the children by respecting their feelings while also requiring them to use prosocial means for dealing with their anger and for regaining some power (Gootman 1993). Caughey (1991) suggests that we allow children to express negative feelings in a safe way, perhaps with creative activities or dramatic play with toys, so that they can come to terms with their reactions to their circumstances and learn that their feelings are not frightening or likely to get out of their control.

You will need to understand that abused children will view their world as dangerous but also you must suggest an alternative point of view (Caughey 1991). You might sit beside them and participate quietly or comment on what they are doing or saying, to help them notice that they are having a positive experience (Caughey 1991). More than most, these children will need empathic responses from educators so that they learn to recognise their own and others' pain; they need attention; and they need to know that they will be safe if they make a mistake (Gootman 1993). Predictable reactions and a safe emotional climate will help formerly hypervigilant children to feel secure again.

Encourage abused children to re-focus on child business

Abuse makes children feel responsible for adults, causing them to sacrifice their personal development and happiness (O'Donnell & Craney 1982). To undo this damage, encourage them to focus on their own growth, without having to worry about the adults in their lives.

Highlight abused children's resilience

While acknowledging the real and profound pain caused by abuse, we must not add to survivors' adjustment difficulties by pitying them and making them feel less than whole or that they cannot cope. People can and do overcome the effects of abuse—sometimes with professional help, but more often with the normal supports of loving friends and family. Therefore, comment on the children's strengths and encourage their efforts to cope. Enhancing abused children's self-esteem is especially important.

Provide child protection training

Personal safety programs are often recommended for preventing children from becoming victims of abuse, although there is little research evidence of the effectiveness of these programs at empowering children to act on the knowledge imparted in the programs (Bevill & Gast 1998), little advice about necessary modifications to ensure age-appropriateness and few guidelines to avoid side-effects such as increased fearfulness in children (Bonner et al. 1992; Jordan 1993).

Nevertheless, protectiveness programs begin by teaching children to recognise their feelings, and to notice when these are telling them that something is wrong. The guiding rule here is: *If you don't feel safe, you aren't safe.* You might ask the children where in their bodies they feel unsafe feelings—say, when they are at the top of a high slippery-dip (or slide); and later teach them the difference between being excited-scared and bad-scared. Children still need to take risks and have fun, and to realise that being good-scared is okay.

A second aspect of protectiveness training relates to the fact that children who have been neglected or abused by a parent will have an impaired attachment to and conflicting emotions about their relationship with their parents, and poor role models for regulating their emotions. So they will need more than the usual coaching to teach them to label emotions and to understand that anger can be resolved without terror.

When adults listen to children about the little things, children will talk with us about the big things. So any chance you get, tell children that *they can tell you anything*, even if it seems awful. Teach them that good secrets always finish: when you keep a secret about someone's birthday present, the secret ends on the birthday. But if someone tells them to keep a secret forever, that means it is a bad secret. Explain that it is safe to tell you any secrets like these.

Another phase of protectiveness training is to help children to make a backup plan for instances when their parents or other caregivers are not available to help them in frightening situations. A formal protectiveness training program gets children to draw around their hand and then on each finger draw or write the names of people they could talk to if they ever needed help. You can then explain that they have to keep persisting, talking to every person on their list in turn if the previous person cannot help them.

Finally, when you see an emergency vehicle racing down a road with its siren blazing, use that as a chance to tell the children that they are allowed to make noise and rush when they feel in danger. They do not have to be polite to someone who is scaring them: they can scream loudly and run away for help.

Use guidance methods of discipline

When you teach children to be considerate instead of compliant, when you are assertive about your needs and teach them to be likewise, and when you listen to and accept their feelings—even the inexplicable ones—you will have inoculated them against being abused. Abuse can occur only within power-based relationships, and if the children do not experience these, they will be able to detect and avoid the abusive use of power over them. By allowing them to think for themselves and be assertive about everyday events, you are giving them skills that they could use not only in these circumstances but when under threat as well.

Support the family

If the welfare agency decides on the basis of your information to investigate the family, you will need the agency's advice about whether you should tell the parents that you have reported your concerns and about how to support the family during the investigation process so that the child is not subjected to further violence or emotional abuse as a result of the disclosure. Even if a family member has been named as the perpetrator, the non-offending adults will need immediate emotional support to help them to cope while the investigation is happening (Briggs 1993). As well, it might be useful to give them some reading material and the names of a parent support group, psychologists or family therapists who could support them during the investigation (Briggs 1993). Your local child welfare agency might be able to recommend some agencies.

If the perpetrator is other than the parents, parents might find the following suggestions helpful:

- Despite their anger—or perhaps because of it—it is not wise for parents to confront the perpetrator themselves. He or she may fool them into believing a plausible explanation of the incidents, which makes it possible for the abuse to continue. Instead, they need to allow child welfare specialists to carry out the investigation.
- The parents must be sure not to blame the children for the disruption that their disclosure causes or for the abuse itself. They might tell the children that, unfortunately, what was done to them happens to lots of children, and so it was not provoked by anything that they did.
- The children will need reassurance that if threats were made, these were not true but were tricks to try to get them to keep the abuse secret.
- Adults must avoid making negative comments about the abuser. This is because when the children know their abuser, they are likely to have both positive and negative feelings about that person. However unlikely it may seem, they generally want the *relationship* with that person to continue but the *abuse* to stop. Explain that the behaviour—not the person—is the problem. The things that the abuser did to them are not fair because children cannot say 'no' to adults who trick them.
- Advise parents to stay close to the children after a disclosure of abuse, while resisting the urge to over-protect or unnecessarily restrict their children. Parents will need to be normally affectionate, so that the children do not assume that their parents no longer love them or are punishing them for being abused or for disclosing the abuse.

- The parents will need to tell their other children what has happened. Because abuse is often multi-victimed, they will need to enquire of siblings whether they too have had a 'worrying secret' or have had someone touching them in 'confusing ways'. Once the parents know that their other children have not been involved, they can tell the children that they can all be safe from now on. They might take this opportunity to educate all their children in self-protection.
- Encourage parents to seek professional help. Many abused children worry whether they have been permanently injured physically, and so they need to be reassured by a thorough medical examination. Meanwhile, parents might need some professional help to overcome their reactions and to get their marriage back in balance, particularly if one parent was the perpetrator of the abuse.

Educate your parent group about child abuse

Raising the issue of abuse with your parent group at times other than crises can highlight how they can keep their children safe, recognise the signs of abuse, and be familiar with reporting procedures.

Children of teen parents

The circumstances of teen parents can compromise their ability to parent their children responsively. Many are living in poverty; some have little family (including partner) support in their child-rearing, while others experience this family intervention as intrusive because of their need to become independent; their immature abstract thinking skills can mean that they fail to anticipate their babies' needs; their developmental egocentrism can cause them to confuse their own needs with their babies' and so misread their child's signals; and many were neglected or abused by their own parents and so have little history of nurturing (Gowen & Nebrig 2002). As a result, their babies' development of an insecure attachment and the parents' difficulty with regulating their emotions can produce behavioural difficulties in their children which, in turn, may be met with punitive responses.

As with other family challenges, your dual role will be to guide the children's behaviour and relate to them in ways that give them experience of receiving supportive and responsive care. Second, you could support the parents in their child-rearing role by, upon invitation, giving direct suggestions on parenting issues or referring them to community agencies that can teach them about child development, offer them support from other teen parents, assist them to further their educational or career planning, and improve their living conditions.

Children whose parents have intellectual disabilities

Children whose parents have intellectual disabilities (or mental retardation, in U.S. terms) are more likely than usual to be living in poverty and lacking in social support (Feldman 1994; Llewellyn 1990, 1994). As a result, the children are at risk of neglect and of receiving insufficient stimulation, with consequent impairment in their development, especially language skills (Llewellyn 1990; Schilling et al. 1982; Tymchuk 1992).

As poverty tends to be long term, the risk to the children is prolonged. Another risk factor for parents with intellectual disabilities is the quality of the parenting which they received as children, particularly if they were placed in foster or institutional care (Llewellyn 1990; Tymchuk 1992) and the fact that during adolescence they are unlikely to have been entrusted with the supervision of children (Schilling et al. 1982) and so will lack experience with and knowledge of children and their development.

Despite these risks of impoverished living circumstances and poor parenting role models, the majority of parents with mild intellectual disabilities are able to parent adequately (Llewellyn 1990). Their parenting skills can be similar to those of non-disabled parents of similar socioeconomic status (Tymchuk 1992), especially when there are two parents and few children in the family.

But when multiple risk factors are present, these parents are likely to need ongoing assistance in their parenting role (Booth & Booth 1995). Specifically, they tend to require the following training and support (Llewellyn et al. 1999; McConnell et al. 1997):

- demonstration of parenting skills so that they can keep their children safe and respond appropriately to the children's changing needs as they develop (Feldman et al. 1989);
- advice about guiding children's behaviour positively, as their concrete thinking and limited decision-making and communication skills can result in impulsive or inflexible responses to their children's behaviours (Llewellyn 1990; Llewellyn & Brigden 1995; Schilling et al. 1982);
- living skills: budgeting and housekeeping so that they can provide adequately for their family;
- self-esteem and assertiveness skills so that they can ask for services that they need and decline those services that they do not want;
- social skills so that they can expand their support network and thus not overtax family and friends or suffer intrusive support from these sources (Booth & Booth 1995);

- access to mainstream services such as parenting groups, as long as these can be adjusted to meet their needs and the parents do not suffer impatience or ridicule from non-disabled group members (Llewellyn 1994; Llewellyn & Brigden 1995); and
- coordinated service provision so that the parents are not subjected to conflicting advice and complex requirements to fulfil in order to receive services (McConnell et al. 1997).

The implication for educators is that when you have a child in your care whose parents have an intellectual disability, you will need to provide your information to them in very concrete terms, bearing in mind their reading and vocabulary skills and difficulties with understanding and learning new concepts (Llewellyn 1995). When you focus on what they want to know and learn, you will motivate them to continue to ask your advice (Llewellyn & Brigden 1995).

You are in an ideal position to refer the family to suitable agencies that could help them, as long as you have their permission to do so. (The exception would be instances of child neglect or abuse, in which case their consent is not required.)

Meanwhile your main role will be to support the children, particularly those who are taking on adult roles at a young age to compensate for their parents' inabilities. Especially as they near school age, the children need to be allowed to talk about their experiences (Ronai 1997). Forcing them to pretend that their family is 'normal' adds another layer of abuse to the challenges of looking after parents while one is still a child.

Children whose parents have a mental illness

Whereas parents with an intellectual disability might not know how best to meet their children's needs, parents with a mental illness might not be aware of their children's needs or might assess these needs on the basis of how they themselves are feeling (Gowen & Nebrig 2002). Furthermore, their care of the children might fluctuate according to the status of their illness, their compliance with medication regimes, and the amount of supports available to them.

The most common mental illness is depression, to which mothers are particularly prone post-natally. Approximately 40–70% experience mild symptoms soon after the birth of their child, with 4% still deeply troubled a year later (Grundy & Roberts, in Field 1989). The incidence is probably higher for parents living in adverse circumstances (Lyons-Ruth et al. 1986). Even if aware of their infants' needs, depressed parents often lack the energy to respond or are emotionally unavailable to their infants, which is likely to be more stressful than physical separation (Field et al. 1986; Goodman & Brumley 1990). As a result, infants as young as three months of age can be irritable, often protest inconsolably, or can display flat affect (Gowen & Nebrig 2002; Zuckerman et al. 1990).

Mothers who are depressed do not always present as sad but rather can be apathetic, resentful of their baby, neglectful, or may handle the child roughly (Cohn & Campbell 1992; Lyons-Ruth 1992). Whatever their actual behaviours, it is clear that the mothers' actions are less responsive than usual to their babies' current mood. In response, the babies often reflect their mothers' depressed state and do not communicate their needs as they develop little expectation of having these met. Thus, it will be important when caring for the babies of depressed mothers that you do not overlook these infants in the false belief that they are simply non-demanding. It can help to assign a primary caregiver who is available as much as possible to give babies of depressed mothers an alternative attachment figure. The babies need to learn to communicate their needs and develop an expectation that these will be responded to. Meanwhile, you might have an opportunity to encourage a depressed parent to secure timely treatment, as untreated maternal depression can have long-lasting effects on children (Field 1992). It can also help if depressed parents can locate some community resources that will improve their quality of life, as the depression can be both a cause and a result of adverse circumstances.

Children of parents who misuse drugs

The two most dangerous drugs for mothers to ingest during pregnancy are nicotine and alcohol. With the rate of births of children with Down syndrome having halved in recent times, fetal alcohol syndrome is now the largest cause of intellectual disability in children, accounting for 10-20% of all instances of intellectual disability (or 1–2 per 1000 live births) (Batshaw & Conlon 1997; Howard et al. 2001). Signs of fetal alcohol syndrome include (Batshaw & Conlon 1997):

- delayed speech, language and motor skills;
- behavioural difficulties;
- below-average height (but normal weight);
- abnormal facial features: small head; short, upturned nose; thin upper lips; flattened philtrum; wide-set eyes; flat midface; and epicanthic folds over the eyes;

- malformations of the outer and middle ear; and
- cardiac, vision and hearing problems.

Lesser effects on development and physical appearance are experienced at lower levels of alcohol intake, when the child's difficulties are usually referred to as 'fetal alcohol effects'. This accounts for three to five live births per 1000.

Exposure to tobacco, marijuana, cocaine, and other illicit drugs in utero results in decreased blood and oxygen reaching the fetus, causing stunted growth and increased risk of miscarriage, premature birth, stillbirth, and sudden infant death (Batshaw & Conlon 1997; Howard et al. 2001).

Meanwhile, some of the developmental effects of alcohol and other drugs can be due not only to the damage to the developing fetus but also to the chaotic home circumstances prevailing when a parent is an addict—not least of which is a lack of supervision and stimulation of the baby, poor prenatal and postnatal care and nutrition, impoverished living circumstances, multiple drug use, and diminished social supports for the family. The spouse abuse and deceit that often accompany a partner's abuse of drugs can reduce the quality of parenting of even the sober parent (Gowen & Nebrig 2002).

Parents are unlikely to admit to their own illicit drug taking or alcoholic drinking patterns but there will be instances when you suspect these to be the cause of their children's disruptive behaviour. The actual behavioural difficulties can be dealt with in any of the ways recommended in earlier chapters; meanwhile, you might be able to entice the parents to gain help for their addiction.

If at any time you suspect that a parent's addiction is leading to neglect of the children, you must report your concerns to your local child welfare agency. (See the earlier section on child abuse.) If able to collaborate with a treating agency, you might plan for increased attendance of the child at your centre while the parent is being treated, so that if the parent relapses into heavy drug use or consumption, sudden changes in child care arrangements are not imposed on children at times when the family is already in crisis (Gowen & Nebrig 2002).

Conclusion

The unfortunate fact is that family risk factors tend to occur in multiples. Poverty, for instance, tends to strain families' internal and external coping resources, limit the solutions that are available to the parents and, in turn, negatively affect the choices they make. Nevertheless, children living in these adverse circumstances will cope as long as their parents can stay in charge and lead the family through its crisis. Although this is more difficult when they are experiencing a constellation of difficulties, parents do not have to have all the answers—or even pretend that they do—but they do need to continue to offer responsive care of the children and to reassure the children that they are working out the issues and will continue to look after themselves and the children while they are determining what needs to be done.

If you become concerned that children's behavioural difficulties are being triggered by family upsets, you could collaborate with the parents to solve the problem (see Chapter 16). Even when parents seem to be acting in ways that are detrimental to their children, you will need to relate to them with the same courtesy as you do all others.

At the same time, your main role as a care provider or educator will be to advocate for the children's needs, supporting the family to meet these and to enact solutions. If you remain concerned about the quality of care that the children are receiving at home, you must act to secure services for the family so that the children can be protected from the serious consequences of neglect or abuse.

Suggested further reading

Some of the following books will be useful for your own background reading; others will be specifically useful to parents.

Death

Fitzgerald, H. (1992). *The grieving child: A parent's guide*. New York: Fireside.
McKissock, D. (1998). *The grief of our children*. Sydney: ABC.
McKissock, M. & McKissock, D. (1995). *Coping with grief*. (3rd ed.) Sydney: ABC.
Wells, R. (1998). *Helping children cope with grief: Facing a death in the family*. London: Sheldon.
Westberg, G.E. (1992). *Good grief*. (rev. ed.) Melbourne: Fortress.

Divorce

Burrett, J. (1999). *But I want to stay with you: Talking with children about separation and divorce*. Sydney: Simon and Schuster.
Teyber, E. (1992). *Helping children cope with divorce*. San Francisco, CA: Jossey-Bass.
Wells, R. (1997). *Helping children cope with divorce*. London: Sheldon.
Weyburne, D. (1999). *What to tell the kids about your divorce*. Oakland, CA: Harbinger.

Stepfamilies

Boyd, H. (1998). *The step-parent's survival guide*. London: Ward Lock.

Hart-Byers, S. (1998). *Secrets of successful step-families*. Port Melbourne: Lothian.

Webber, R. (1994). *Living in a step-family*. (2nd ed.) Melbourne: A.C.E.R.

Spouse abuse

Brinegar, J. (1992). *Breaking free from domestic violence*. Center City, MN: CompCare Publishers.

Evans, P. (1996). *The verbally abusive relationship: How to recognize it and how to respond*. (2nd ed.) Holbrook, MA: Adams Media Corporation.

Marecek, M. (1993). *Breaking free from partner abuse: Voices of battered women caught in the cycle of domestic violence*. Buena Park, CA: Morning Glory Press.

Child abuse

Adams, C. & Fay, J. (1992). *Helping your child recover from sexual abuse*. Seattle, WA: University of Washington Press.

Bass, E. & Davis, L. (1993). *Beginning to heal: A first guide for female survivors of child sexual abuse*. London: Vermilion.

Briggs, F. (1993). *Why my child?: Supporting the families of victims of child sexual abuse*. Sydney: Allen and Unwin.

Briggs, F. & McVeity, M. (2000). *Teaching children to protect themselves*. Sydney: Allen and Unwin.

Davis, L. (1991). *Allies in healing: When the person you love was sexually abused as a child*. New York: Harper Perennial.

Hunter, M. (1990). *Abused boys: The neglected victims of sexual abuse*. New York: Fawcett Columbine.

Lew, M. (1990). *Victims no longer: A guide for men recovering from sexual child abuse*. London: Cedar.

Sonkin, D.J. (1998). *Wounded boys; heroic men: A man's guide to recovering from child abuse*. Holbrook, MA: Adams Media Corporation.

Part Five

●●

Caring for adults

Positive and healthy organizational climates are characterized by high energy, openness, trust, a collective sense of efficacy, and a shared vision.

Jorde-Bloom (1988: 5)

The adults in child care or preschool centres are like the hub of a wheel. You form the core, with your relationships with children, parents, the wider community, and your governing bodies being the spokes. Each spoke strengthens the wheel—but it is the core that shapes all the other aspects of the centre: its atmosphere, warmth of relationships, and the quality of the program.

Increasingly, the care and education of young children is seen to be a mutual concern of their parents and caregiver-teachers. In order to feel empowered to fulfil their respective roles, both partners to this relationship will need support and resources.

Therefore, in this section, I examine some of the issues that affect your ability to experience satisfaction in your work and to discharge your responsibilities in the best way you know how. This requires that you have access to support, as your role in caring for and educating young children is a demanding and complex one—and whenever demands are high, supports necessarily must be high also. Among other things, this involves recruiting the support of parents, which is more likely when you can appreciate their perspective and harness their expertise in caring for their children. The final chapter on writing a discipline policy is aimed at formalising some of those supports through a process of collaboration with colleagues and parents to define practices that will be effective, ethical and widely endorsed by all stakeholders.

15

●●

Supporting staff

The teachers of our children deserve the same quality of treatment that we expect them to offer our children.

Hilliard (1985: 22)

It is not the purpose of this chapter to detail all that is involved in supporting educators in early childhood centres. That would be too large a task for a single chapter. However, this chapter will examine the types of supports that staff can require to frame a workable system for guiding children's behaviour.

Provide conducive working conditions

Children—particularly the very young—are highly sensitive to the morale of the people around them (Smith 1990). Therefore, the working conditions in a centre directly affect the children as well as the adults who work there (Doherty-Derkowski 1995; Smith 1990). Thus, safeguarding your working conditions is as much for the children's benefit as your own.

Provide adequate staffing

Staffing levels and staff qualifications are two of the most crucial aspects in determining the quality of care children receive—as high adult-child ratios permit close interactions between adults and children (Arthur et al. 1996; Phillips & Howes 1987). Meanwhile, staff with extensive training are more likely to engage positively and be less restrictive with children (Howes 1983b). Thus, not only does adequate staffing benefit caregivers: it also supports the children.

Avoid overload

When individuals feel out of control, their natural tendency is to try harder to take control, both over themselves and others. In care and teaching professions, stressed adults become more concerned with ensuring their own survival than with safeguarding children's needs (Lewis 1997). The result is that exhausted or burnt out workers are more likely to supervise children from a distance, rather than relating to them personally, and tend to focus on controlling children rather than using more responsive management strategies (Lambert 1994; Lewis 1997).

As well, exhausted staff tend to adopt a clinical attitude to children, whereby they blame individual children for disruptive acts and even attempt to diagnose what is 'wrong' with the children, rather than looking at the circumstances that might be provoking those disruptions (Lambert 1994). Therefore, both for the direct effects on adults' wellbeing and for the indirect effects that worker stress can have on the quality of care being delivered to the children, centre management must take active steps to avoid overloading staff.

Many aspects of working with groups of children can contribute to overload in adults. The work is *multi-dimensional*, which is to say that many different people with different interests and abilities are sharing the same space; many things are happening *simultaneously*; and events can unfold rapidly and unpredictably, demanding *immediate* responses (Doyle 1986). Meanwhile, all your responses are public, being witnessed by other children, colleagues and visitors to the centre. This has two effects: first, that one child's disruptive behaviour can become contagious—that is, other children might join in; and, second, that any action that you take tells onlookers (both adults and children) about your skills and about how safe they are in the centre. This sheer complexity is an everyday challenge that needs careful managing if overload or burnout are to be avoided.

It is my observation that those caregivers who are most capable and those who seem to be coping best—even if already overworked—are the ones to be allocated the most demanding children. Obviously, skilled people need to be dealing with the children who require the most expertise, but we risk burning out good staff if they are not relieved of other commitments when new ones are added.

It is also important to minimise unnecessary tasks or to streamline those that are compulsory. As one of many examples, in one of the centres observed during my research into child (day) care centres, children were required to remove their shoes whenever they entered the sandpit and then put them on again whenever they left (Porter 1999b). Picture the amount of work this created as staff had to assist those children who could not don shoes independently!

It is thus important that centre management listen to feedback from staff about unnecessary tasks, as if these consume the few precious minutes that are free for relating with children, the children will necessarily receive less care. All staff need to keep in mind that procedures are there to serve you, rather than your being a servant to them.

Safeguard caregivers' time off

There needs to be climate in any centre whereby staff are graciously afforded the breaks they need to recoup their energies. Each centre needs a calm and pleasant area to which caregivers can withdraw, rather than sitting in rooms little bigger than closets, cluttered by the accoutrements of their work. If caregivers' breaks are stress-ridden, their subsequent care of the children may suffer.

Provide ample planning and evaluation time

There need to be systems in place to ensure that the program runs efficiently and effectively so that it meets the needs and desires of children, parents and staff (Sebastian 1989; Simons 1986). There are many threats to the sanctity of planning time, but centre managers and staff will need to insist on time to plan for meeting these needs and regularly reviewing the wider program.

Offer regular staff training

In addition to all your other expertise, training about the theories that govern your disciplinary practices is fundamental because, if left having to make moment-by-moment decisions, you will be working too hard. This will inevitably result in exhaustion and poorer decisions than you might otherwise make. Instead, if you can draw on a clear rationale for your practices, each decision will be more automatic. In turn, it is likely to be more effective, and less stressful for you.

Successful staff development will renew your enthusiasm for your work, improve your confidence in your abilities, and allow you to continue to grow professionally (Greenman & Stonehouse 1997). Caregivers with more training tend to be less authoritarian in their discipline (Arnett 1989), which reinforces the importance of training in a guidance approach.

A naturalistic form of staff training is the supervision of less experienced staff. However, supervisors generally receive very little training for this role and, consequently, often experience anxiety about it—so they too need some support in this task (Caruso 1991). Other forms of staff development include collecting a staff library of books and other resources for caregivers to access; arranging staff exchanges with other centres; and presenting workshops by staff from other centres or community specialists (Abbott-Shim 1990). Hired consultants are the most expensive option but when their input can be especially tailored to your centre's needs, the training can be most effective.

The most important outcome of training is to empower caregivers to reflect on their practices, questioning their underlying values, beliefs and assumptions which otherwise might have been taken for granted (Roth 1989; Smyth 1989). Another byproduct will be that staff can become less isolated from other professionals, allowing for subsequent exchanges of ideas outside of formal training sessions.

Facilitate collegial support

Collegiality is the extent to which staff support and trust each other and are friendly and caring towards each other (Jorde-Bloom 1988). If you keep pouring out without topping up your emotional store, you will burn out, like the element of a kettle when water is poured out and not topped-up again. Therefore, the support from other members of your staff team can make a difference to how well you are able to function and how well you feel physically and emotionally.

New workers are particularly likely to feel overwhelmed by the responsibility of caring for young children, uncertain of how their ideas will be accepted by more experienced staff, and anxious about responding to children's inconsiderate or disruptive behaviour (Brand 1990; Fleet & Clyde 1993). With emotional, practical and professional support from colleagues and a willingness to grow and learn, however, new workers can move from 'survival mode' to a consolidation or mastery stage in which they develop confidence and autonomy as professionals (Brand 1990; Clyde 1988; Fleet & Clyde 1993).

Give emotional support

When a member of staff is confronting a particularly chronic or challenging behavioural difficulty with any of the children, other staff members need to give both practical and moral support, not as a favour but as a matter of course (Rogers 1994). This might even mean that staffing schedules will have to be adjusted until the child's behaviour settles and the extra demands on the primary caregiver have decreased.

Develop teamwork

The various staff members in your centre will warm to different children, will not find the same behaviours annoying and will not have exactly the same disciplinary approaches. You can still work as a team, however, without being identical. Successful teamwork can mean harnessing each person's strengths and interests. It can also mean that when one of the team becomes irritated by a particular behaviour, he or she can ask a colleague to take over. This is not an admission of defeat but a recognition that it is okay to look after yourself. It communicates that you are still in command and are not being rescued, but merely supported.

Although guidance approaches do not require consistency to be effective, repeated practice will help children to learn self-control quickly (see Chapter 9). Therefore, when one caregiver is occupied for a prolonged period with a disruptive child, others will need to take over the routine tasks that must continue. This is aided when staff can be flexible about their roles but also means that, when staff simply are not available to deal at length with a disruption, a less labour-intensive approach must be used (again, see Chapters 9 and 10).

Exercise leadership

Your team leader, director or centre owner needs to provide leadership for the whole staff team. But this is not to say that the centre director needs to be a boss. Whereas a boss gains compliance through having power over others, a leader invites cooperation—and this is willingly given because others recognise the leader's skills and expertise.

Leadership involves vision and influence (Rodd 1996). A team leader needs to be able to enthuse all the staff to share a common vision of the purpose of the centre; to listen to their ideas for innovations in order that the program responds to children's and parents' changing needs (Broinowski 1994); be skilful at developing a team culture, clear goals and objectives; and have good communication skills (Billman 1995). Team leaders need to be able to delegate duties that are more appropriately done by someone else (Jorde-Bloom 1988) and give educators professional autonomy, while maintaining standards through supervision and program evaluation (Billman 1995). At the same time, leaders need to be carry out their administrative functions efficiently, thus supporting other members of staff in their respective roles (Billman 1995).

Practise consultation

Caregivers are more likely to feel valued when the centre director trusts other members of staff and parents to make valuable contributions and wise decisions, rather than imposing decisions on them with little consultation (Bloom 1982; Clyde 1988; Greenman & Stonehouse 1997). Staff are certain to become discouraged if their ideas for innovations and improvements are constantly squashed in a centre which dismisses suggestions with a claim that, 'We have always done it this way'. Centres that survive—and retain skilled staff—will be those that are open to new ideas and are willing to take risks in an effort to respond to the changing needs of caregivers, parents and children.

Recognise the efforts of staff

Although early childhood workers are acknowledged to be underpaid and a centre is unlikely to be able to pay above-average wages, staff will feel less dissatisfied if they believe that their own centre's policies are fair and if they feel that their skills are not being taken for granted by management. The occasional social gathering or positive comment about their work can at least partly compensate for the lack of monetary rewards.

Seek outside guidance

Caregivers cannot be expected to continue dealing without supports with behaviours that are not responding to their best preventive and interventive methods. With respect to intractable behavioural difficulties, a key ethical principle is that children and families have a right to competent service. At times, this will mean drawing on outside expertise.

Consult with parents

When children are behaving disruptively in your centre, there will come a time when you must advise their parents. As mentioned in the next chapter, it will be important that you convey the message that you expect to solve centre-based problems within the centre and so do not need the parents to discipline the child at home over issues that arise when in your care. The purposes of advising parents are simply that they have a right to be informed, and to call on their expertise and advice about how you might respond. More is said about this in Chapter 16.

Refer to specialists

When a child's behaviour is proving intractable, once you have parental permission, you must refer the child to a specialist. It is no admission of defeat to call in outside specialists: it would be negligent to continue to deal with something that is beyond your previous experience and limits of expertise.

To that end, it can be useful to be aware of a paediatric specialists in a range of fields, how parents can contact these, and the costs and waiting periods involved. Your parent group can be a useful fund of knowledge here. By asking them which practitioners they have used and can recommend, you can build up a list of practitioners in various fields: paediatricians, podiatrists, physiotherapists, chiropractors, psychologists, paediatric dentists, speech pathologists, naturopaths, and so on, whose names you could give to parents when a need arises.

Conclusion

With leadership and commitment, a staff team can create a positive climate in the centre—a tone which supports the children, parents and staff who live and work there (Jorde-Bloom 1988). A benefit of meeting the needs of staff is that centres are likely to reduce the usually high rate of staff turnover experienced in the early childhood sector—which averages 15-30% (Bloom 1982). High staff turnover directly affects the rate of interaction between staff and children, the children's attachment to their caregiver-teachers, and the children's language development (Doherty-Derkowski 1995). It also stresses their caregivers.

When staff are treated with respect and valued for their contributions, it is easier for them to treat children with respect, relate to them with interest and warmth, guide rather than control them, respond to them individually rather than as a group, and encourage them to be active in their learning. The more engaged caregivers are with the children, the more likely it is that their work will be effective and their relationship with the children will uplift their own spirits.

Suggested further reading

Centre directors might find some useful ideas in:
Broinowski, I. (1994). *Managing child care centres*. Melbourne: TAFE Publications.

The following handbook might be of interest to staff who are feeling exhausted by their work:
Lambert, B. (1994). *Beating burnout: A multi-dimensional perspective*. AECA Resource Book Series, 1 (2). Watson, ACT: Australian Early Childhood Association.

16

Solving problems in collaboration with parents

> *Child care professionals have learned that children are best served when providers have some understanding of the children's primary world at home. They also know that a spirit of partnership with parents promotes a higher quality of child care and that maintaining open lines of communication is an important means to that end.*
>
> KLEINMAN (1988: XI)

This chapter will not cover all aspects of collaborating with parents: like the rest of this book, its focus will remain on working with parents when a concern has arisen about their child's behaviour. It will begin by focusing on the style of your interactions—that is, how you relate to parents—and then move on to examining how to solve problems in collaboration with them.

Rationale for parental collaboration

The drive towards parental collaboration is based on a number of assumptions at the heart of which is a belief that a partnership with parents is in their child's best interests (Sebastian 1989: 77):

- parents have the most important and enduring relationship with their children;

- children learn more from their home environment than from any other setting;
- parents' involvement in their child's education contributes to children's positive attitudes to learning and to themselves as learners (Raban 1997);
- parental involvement in their child's educational or care setting promotes mutual respect and understanding between the home and the centre;
- parents can make valuable contributions to caregivers' knowledge of children by passing on their expertise about their own children, their informed observations of their children over a long period of time and in many circumstances, knowledge of their children's needs, and their skill in reading and responding to their children's cues; and
- accountability is more open when parents are involved in their child's program.

However, these reasons focus on the benefits for children alone, when an emerging emphasis in early childhood education is that caregiver-educators have a role in supporting parents and the wider community, as well as meeting children's needs directly. This family- and community-centred view of services upholds that the interests of children are best met by promoting the whole family's healthy functioning and maintaining the parents' confidence in their ability to care for their children. This goal of supporting families, then, becomes a second major rationale for collaborating with parents.

A collaborative style

Parents' participation in their child's education does not necessarily mean day-to-day involvement in a centre (Arthur et al. 1996). As many parents use early childhood services because they are employed or are already balancing the complex demands of their parenting and other roles, pressure to participate intensively can inadvertently add to the strains that they already experience (Sebastian 1989).

Instead, collaboration is a philosophical stance that implies a shared responsibility for the care and education of young children. This collaborative frame of mind is underpinned by six fundamental values: respect, humanness, empowerment, positivity, sensitivity and responsiveness.

Respect

Naturally, most of us find it easiest to accept families whose backgrounds are similar to our own (Galinsky 1990). But the result is that the families who are least well equipped to care for their children, are the least likely to receive the support they need (Arthur et al. 1996; Galinsky 1988). So, although you cannot expect yourself to like every parent, you can respect them for their efforts to bring up their children, recognising that they want the best for their children and have skills and expertise (Gartrell 1998).

Sometimes, however, some widespread myths about families can interfere with forming respectful relationships with those who depart from the 'ideal' picture of the nuclear family with its two adults and their two biological children. These myths are so commonplace that most of us do not even know that they are fallacies. For instance, you might not be aware of the following facts.

- In Victoria, Australia, the rate of single-parent households with dependent children is the same today (16.6%) as it was in 1890 (16.7%). Throughout the intervening century, many fathers left their families during the Depressions in search of work or went to war, in both cases sometimes not returning (McDonald 1993). In the U.S. 28% to 34% of white children born between 1920 and 1960 lived with one or no biological parents, with the figure for black children for roughly the same era being 55% to 60% (Hernandez 1994, in Hanson & Carta 1995). Hanson and Carta predicted that in the period from 1980 these figures could be expected to rise to 50% for white children and 80% for black children.

- The vast majority of today's single parents were in a stable relationship that subsequently disintegrated: they did not set out to be single parents. Whereas in 1971, one in four Australian women had a child before her 20th birthday, by 1990, this figure decreased to one in ten.

- Although divorce is clearly far more common today than ever before, nevertheless life expectancy has increased, and so marriages are today *more* likely to last in excess of 30 years than they were a century ago (McDonald 1993).

- Marital separation does not trouble children as much as living in a conflict-ridden intact family (Burns & Goodnow 1985). If separation does trouble them, this is usually because the separation has not ended the parents' conflict or because it has exacerbated the family's already-impoverished living circumstances.

- The rate of stepfamilies is the same now as it was in the 16th and 17th centuries (Whelan & Kelly 1986). Of course, stepfamily establishment these days usually follows divorce whereas in the past it followed the death of a spouse. Although this difference may change its psychological impact, nevertheless these figures tell us that stepfamilies are not a new family form.

- Throughout history, women have always worked: because they were too poor to do otherwise, to supplement the family income during Depression years, or while men were away at wars. The only exception was the decade of the 1950s when women left the work force as the men returned from World War Two, but this decade is held up today as the norm when in fact it was the exception.

Put together, these facts mean that departures from the idealised 'nuclear' family are not new. This recognition allows us to acknowledge that many types of families can bring up happy children, as long as they have external supports for doing so.

Nevertheless, there are parents whose skills *are* difficult to respect. In these cases, it is worth keeping in mind the following advice (Gowen & Nebrig 2002).

- Some parents who use less-than-ideal parenting practices (such as spanking) nevertheless might do so out of a well-intentioned wish, say, to keep their children safe or to teach them how to behave. In these cases, when the issue comes up in conversation or you observe them using a detrimental practice while they are at your centre, you could ask if they would like to try a new technique that will work just as well but without the disadvantages of their present approach.
- Parents who appear to be parenting poorly often themselves received inadequate care as children. In turn, their troubled childhoods can cause them to feel unworthy and so they will be very sensitive to any criticism of them now.
- In turn, their sense of unworthiness can lead to poor decisions about their use of drugs or choice of life partner, sometimes choosing and then remaining with spouses (de facto or married) who belittle or abuse them further. These problems, in turn, cause a deterioration in their parenting capacities.

Parents who did not experience sensitive and responsive relationships through their formative years and who lack support now will have great difficulty providing sensitive care for their children. Although your role will not be a therapeutic one for these parents, you can be sure that you are reliable and uncritical of them so that they experience receiving support from you. You might be able to assist parents to gain new information or to receive external support to empower them to make changes that would improve their child's circumstances.

Meanwhile respect does not mean that you must agree with them, but simply that you recognise their values, the circumstances they are experiencing (Caughey 1991), and the fact that they can survive crises and manage their challenging family situation (Rosenthal & Sawyers 1996). It might be helpful to keep in mind that people do the best they can in the circumstances that confront them.

Remember also that parents can seem to be less competent than they actually are, because you observe them interacting with their children during their most stressful times of the day—at drop-off and pick-up of their children, when strain and exhaustion are likeliest to show.

Humanness

Most parents will want an emotionally rich relationship with centre staff, rather than formal and distant interactions. However, this is not the same as being friends, because friendship has no agenda whereas your relationship with parents has a particular purpose and, second, being paid to deliver a service renders it a non-friendship. Therefore, friendliness must be balanced with limits on your professional relationships, lest parents become too reliant on you and you become overwhelmed with excessive demands.

Empowerment

In order to function effectively as the hub or key decision-makers in their families, parents need to feel that they have something valuable to contribute. This belief is sometimes termed 'empowerment'. To experience confidence in themselves, parents need (Turnbull & Turnbull 1997):

- recognition of their skills;
- encouragement to contribute to their child's care and to decision-making;
- information about their options;
- a sense of control over their options; and
- support (both formal and informal) for their family leadership role.

Empowerment is mutual, of course. By harnessing parents' expertise and intimate knowledge of their child, you gain information that helps you to provide a better service to the child and family and are more likely to feel assured of the parents' support for your efforts.

Positivity

Positivity involves thinking the best about children's and families' strengths, your own skills and the possibility for improving children's circumstances. At the same time, positivity must be balanced with realism: it is no kindness to parents to withhold information about their child's difficulties out of a misguided wish to shield them or to protect yourself from confronting them with unpleasant information.

Sensitivity

When collaborating with families, it is important to be sensitive to *their circumstances* as these will affect what energies they have available to support their children's care. If the parents are in the process of separating or of establishing a stepfamily, or if one adult is parenting alone, there may be little surplus energy left to devote to collaborating with you over their child's difficulties at your centre.

Such demands can fluctuate from time to time, whereas families who are living in poverty frequently must endure its many disadvantages in the long term. When added to this, the parents themselves have a disability, come from a non-majority culture, or otherwise lack support from the wider community, their participation can be severely compromised as they focus instead on personal and family survival.

A second aspect of sensitivity involves listening to *parents' perspective on using child care*. Most will feel positively about your nurturing relationship with their child and will be satisfied with the quality of care that their child receives but, at the same time, many feel ambivalent about the restricted care options that are available to them and would prefer other forms of care if these were accessible and affordable (Galinsky 1989, 1990).

A third aspect of sensitivity is *listening to parents' aspirations* for their son or daughter: what do they want their child to be gaining from your program? Various parents will have differing aims for their child's participation. Those who are employed but return to work reluctantly are likely to want child care to mirror the nurturing relationships they would prefer to be providing at home (Larner & Phillips 1994). They might try to minimise the amount of time that their child spends in care and so deliver him or her at the latest moment, leaving little time for informal conferences with staff or a relaxed parting from their child. These parents might leave detailed instructions about how they want you to care for their child, and could appear to be very demanding of you (Larner & Phillips 1994).

In contrast, those parents who return to the work force for their own occupational satisfaction are more likely to regard child care as a valuable educational experience and so will be seeking a placement that supplements or complements the experiences that they can offer at home (Larner & Phillips 1994). These parents might question you about the ratio of adults to children, the training and experience of staff in your centre and details of your program. They could be especially focused on outcomes, and question the value of a play-based program if they are unaware of its educational aims. As consumers of an expensive and important service, parents would be irresponsible if they did not closely question what you offer their child and how you deliver your service (Greenman & Stonehouse 1997) so you need not take their questions as challenging your expertise but as requests for information and reassurance.

A fourth aspect to which you will need to be sensitive is *parents' emotions about separation* from their child. Even when the parents are highly motivated to return to the work force, their use of day care still causes them conflict, guilt and sadness (Rolfe et al. 1991). Their subsequent adjustment to being parted from their child is a highly personal and individual process, punctuated with feelings of chronic sadness that can take some months to resolve (Rolfe et al. 1991). Regardless of the quality of the program, this process of grieving and adjusting is common, although parents' feelings are more readily resolved when they feel safe about the quality of care their child is receiving (Larner & Phillips 1994).

Many parents are also acutely aware of their own vulnerability, brought about by their reliance on the ongoing quality of the program that you provide their child. They are painfully aware that they cannot anticipate problems that might arise after they have enrolled their child in your centre (Larner & Phillips 1994). Staff changes, the changing needs of a growing child, and other unforseen changes can neither be anticipated nor guarded against.

On the other hand, although sensitivity and empathy towards families are clearly beneficial, you must avoid feeling sympathy for those in unfortunate circumstances. Pity does not give families confidence in their own ability to overcome adversity and can overwhelm you with 'compassion fatigue' and result in burn out.

Responsiveness

Having been sensitive to parents' and children's needs, responsiveness involves providing, arranging for or recommending services that can help families to meet these needs. Responsiveness can also mean not imposing services that parents do not want.

Nevertheless, although responding to families' requests is important, as with the other aspects of family-centredness, this too can be overdone. You cannot be expected to violate your professional principles (see p. 218) and too much helpfulness can unwittingly undermine parents, creating dependence on outsiders and reducing their confidence in their ability to solve their own problems.

Communicating with parents

There are many occasions when you can exchange information with parents. These include day-to-day informal contacts at drop off and pick-up times; brochures and other written information about the centre's policies and procedures; posters or bulletin boards explaining the rationale of various activities; newsletters; and formal meetings at enrolment, to solve problems or to review children's programs. Of these, problem-solving meetings are likely to be the most personally challenging for you.

Communication with parents will require the same three communication skills that are necessary for working with children—namely, listening, being assertive and solving problems collaboratively. As discussed in Chapter 7, each of these is best employed according to who is feeling concern at the time:

- when parents are concerned, you will need to listen;
- when you are disturbed by someone else's actions, you need to be assertive about the effect the action has on you (followed by listening for their reaction)—bearing in mind that it can avoid defensiveness to use an empathic assertive statement whereby you reflect the other person's concerns, state your alternative perspective, and then ask how the two can be reconciled (Jakubowski & Lange 1978); and
- when you both are being inconvenienced by an issue, you will each need to be assertive, listen to each other, and then solve the problem jointly. This entails defining the problem, listing potential solutions, selecting one of these, implementing it, and then checking that the solution is achieving the desired outcome.

Whichever form your communication takes, it will be important to keep in mind that your goal is not to reform families or ensure that parents use the same behavioural guidance approach as yourself. Remember from Chapter 9 that consistency is unnecessary, as children are wise enough to tune into the various expectations of differing adults and settings and can adjust accordingly—although obviously the more practice they get across settings at behaving thoughtfully, the more quickly they will learn to do so. However, you cannot control the home setting: all you can affect is how you respond to the child in your centre.

Routine communication

Children are more likely to settle in a centre when they know their parents and care staff support and value each other's contributions. To that end, the centre will need procedures for day-to-day communication with parents and for regular updates about children's progress (NAEYC 1984).

However, there is a fine line between conveying a 'holier than thou' attitude and having a 'jollier than thou' tone in the likes of newsletters or notes home to parents. I find the 'hale and hearty' tone of many of these communications patronising. On the one hand, it can seem as if we are jollying parents along, almost as if they were young children themselves. On the other, judging parents—say, by praising them for attending a recent function at the centre—implies that you are the expert and you know best how they should be bringing up their children. Instead, when you keep in mind that you and the parents are jointly working in their child's interests, you will convey in a respectful tone the information that they need to know in order to fulfil their part of that partnership.

Collaborating to resolve disruptive behaviours

When children's behaviour is disrupting others, you will need to inform parents of their child's behaviour, as they have a right to be informed. However, you must balance supplying enough information with providing a surfeit, such that the parents start to avoid conversations with you out of fear of hearing yet another report of their child's disruptiveness.

Furthermore, it is important when talking about problems with parents that you make it clear that you are merely keeping them informed, rather than expecting them to solve the problem for you or to punish the child at home for behaviour displayed at the centre. You need to make it clear that you are looking for a solution rather than seeking to blame or shame the child.

It will help two parent-families if you can speak with both parents about your concerns. If this cannot be arranged, you could tape your conversation so that the parent who could not attend can at least listen to the taped conversation later. You will need to pass on the invitation for that parent to contact you with any questions that arise from hearing the tape.

Preparation

It should first be said that problem-solving meetings will be much more productive when you have maintained ongoing contact with parents over positive and interesting things their son or daughter has been doing in the centre.

Whether a meeting is designed to introduce parents to the centre, routinely review a child's response to the program or solve a problem that has arisen, you will need to plan ahead for your conversation with parents.

Being prepared for problem-solving meetings requires that you gather examples of the child's behaviours that are causing concern and are clear about the aims of the meeting so that you can be equally clear when the meeting has achieved its purpose.

If you are wanting to recommend a specialist assessment for a child with behavioural or other difficulties, before the meeting, ensure that you have updated your knowledge of which agencies are available to provide the type of service the child requires. This information will include waiting times, costs and contact phone numbers. The more specific your information can be, the easier it will be for the parents to follow up your concerns promptly.

Listen to parents

The doctrine of honouring diversity in children extends to their families as well. In multicultural societies, it is not possible, nor even desirable, to approach every parent in the same way (a'Beckett 1988). Whether parents come from a different culture from your own, have a son or daughter with a disability, have a gifted child or in any other way have different needs from the usual, you will need to avoid stereotypes about what they may be experiencing and instead *listen* to their aspirations for their child and their preferred method of responding to difficulties. In terms of the focus of this book on guiding children's behaviour, this information will ensure that any disciplinary plan that is devised does not violate the family's values.

Delivering sensitive information

There will be occasions when you have concerns about a child's behaviour and need to convey these to his or her parents. Earlier I noted that it is important to approach parents positively but realistically. When conveying potentially upsetting information about children to their parents, Ginott (1972: 277–278) cautions:

> *When a teacher talks to parents about their children, he [or she] inevitably intrudes on family dreams . . . What the teacher says about the child touches on deep feelings and hidden fantasies. A concerned teacher is aware of the impact of his [or her] words. He [or she] consciously avoids comments that may casually kill dreams.*

This means that you will need to plan sufficient time to make parents feel comfortable, to discuss your concerns and listen to the parents' reactions (Abbott & Gold 1991). Their first reaction to a suggestion of a difficulty can be anger that they inadvertently direct at you, when instead its real source is their overwhelming worry for their child. At these times, it pays to listen and reflect their fears before gently moving them towards developing a plan to identify and respond to the child's needs.

Seek parents' advice

When attempting to resolve a behavioural or other difficulty of a child in your centre, it is wise not to give the parents advice about how to solve the problem, as dispensing solutions is an exercise of power and, as Bailey (1987) observes, is something done *for* families rather than *with* them. Instead, you can invite the parents to help you solve the problem. Perhaps you could ask them about similar behaviours that have presented at home, how the parents have responded to these, and what effect those measures have had on the behaviour.

Find a solution

Having generated some potential solutions through your discussion thus far with parents, using the collaborative problem-solving steps that were outlined in Chapter 7, together you can plan a solution on the basis of (Heath 1994):

- the parents' and your own overall aspirations for the child;
- the types of solutions that are possible in the circumstances;
- information about what has worked or failed in the past either at home or in the centre;
- relevant characteristics of the child—such as his or her interests, temperament, age or size (as this affects the child's ability to dominate his or her peers, for instance); and
- the needs of surrounding children and adults so that your joint solution is compatible with your broader educational goals for the child and satisfies the needs of all those involved.

If the parents want you to solve a difficulty in a way that contradicts your professional judgment about best practice, it will not be possible to follow their advice because, although a fundamental principle of a pluralistic service is to respect parents' views, educators must also respect their own professional expertise (Powell 1994). However, if you argue against their suggestion, you might undermine them. Explaining the rationale of your approach is one option, but in so doing you cannot attempt to change parents' values (Powell 1994). Perhaps parents can select another service that more closely reflects their values but, in reality, few options can be available so persistent disagreement can be difficult to resolve.

Referral

If a child's behaviour is of serious concern and you feel the need for consultation with an outside specialist, you will of course require parental consent to make a referral. At this stage, it will not be your task to diagnose what is causing the child's behaviour, but simply to recommend a specialist assessment. If this assessment uncovers a behavioural or other difficulty, the parents might react in a range of ways reported in Chapter 13, at which time it can be important for you to provide a listening ear (when available) to support them as they focus their efforts on assisting their child.

A second instance where referral to an outside agency can be called for is when the parents have need for support that is beyond your capacity to provide. In line with the adage that the most troubled parents are usually the most isolated, you might be able to support the parents—and thus indirectly improve their child's circumstances—by helping isolated parents to locate some social supports. This might comprise formal service agencies, or could just involve linking families within your centre, perhaps by suggesting that a parent invite a friend of their child home, which gives the child social contact and puts the two sets of parents in contact with each other.

Responding to parental complaints

A second scenario is when parents come to you with complaints about the management of their child's behaviour in your centre. On these occasions, it can help to keep in mind that both of you want what is best for their child—even when you have differing ideas about how to achieve this. This means that, regardless of their manner, the questions that parents ask and the demands they make need to be met with courtesy. Even those 'difficult' parents are not being demanding just to make you jump through hoops: they both *need* and have a *right* to ask questions.

Your first task when parents come to you with a complaint will be to *listen*. You will need to reflect what they are saying and acknowledge how they are feeling.

However, there will be occasions when parents are belligerent, uncooperative, abusive or otherwise disrespectful or overpowering (Boutte et al. 1992). Although at first glance these behaviours can intimidate you, generally the parents feel that they have a valid reason for their frustrations. It can help to keep in mind that their anger is not actually directed at you personally but at a situation in which they feel powerless. Nevertheless, although you must listen to their complaint, if parents are expressing themselves offensively, it is perfectly appropriate to ask them to moderate their language. Having reflected their feelings, you might have to add an assertive statement such as, 'I accept that you are angry that Simon was sent to sit by himself to calm down, although I do not like how you are saying it'. As children, many parents were let down or disappointed by those on whom they relied and as a result expect you to give up on them too, in which case it will be important for you not to succumb to your very natural emotional reactions to their anger (Gowen & Nebrig 2002).

The next step is to state that you share a common interest—namely, providing the best possible care for their child. You might re-focus the discussion on the topic of how to do so: 'I wonder how we could ensure that in future he can calm down without having to go to the quiet corner to do it'.

Another possibility is to ask for a break to consider the issue that is concerning the parents. If you give yourself time to evaluate parents' complaints, it is less likely that you will become defensive or apologetic about them (Heath 1994). Take the information, offer to think about it or gather more facts from another member of staff about the incident in question, and agree to get back to the parents. Building in a delay in this way will also give the parents time to cool down. They will not be able to listen to even the most reasonable explanation while they are angry (Stanley 1996). A postponement will also avoid having the conflict escalate and will keep you safe from physical abuse or intimidation.

Complaints from third parties

Parents whose children are being victimised repeatedly by another child have grounds for protest about this. Even when their own child is not a direct recipient of aggressive behaviour, they can still have legitimate concerns about how much time a troublesome child is detracting from the care that is available to their own son or daughter.

The politics of behaviour management are actually more complex than the practice itself. The issue of how much you should disclose about the behaviour of another child is delicate and needs to be decided on a case-by-case basis. Giving the wider parent group too much information could create unnecessary anxiety or be construed as a tacit invitation for protests; conversely, if you do not discuss the issue, some parents might feel that you are not receptive to their legitimate concerns. You must also have a view to maintaining confidentiality about the perpetrator and his or her family.

Obviously, the dilemma will be solved if the child's offensive behaviour can be improved; if it cannot, there is some argument for advising his or her parents that your setting is not meeting the child's needs, and suggesting that instead a smaller, more intimate arrangement—such as family day care—could better suit the child while also preventing the repeated victimisation and intimidation of surrounding children. As mentioned in Chapter 1, it is unjust to allow the needs of one child to eclipse the needs of others.

Preparing parents for transitions

If you have been working successfully for some time with parents to resolve an issue about their child, they may have become reliant on you. Parents are vulnerable and rely heavily on the close and trusting relationship they develop with their child's caregivers, and so moving on to another group can be a traumatic time for them as well as for their child. Therefore, you will need to give extra support to both children and their parents as they prepare to move to another section of your centre or on to school.

Conclusion

Collaboration with parents over behavioural issues will not occur by accident: you will need to plan for it, taking into account the differing availability of families to participate in problem solving. Means of collaborating with parents will need to be written into your centre's policy and you may benefit from additional training in the skills required to work jointly with parents.

Suggested further reading

Stonehouse, A. (1994). *How does it feel?: Child care from a parent's perspective.* Canberra, ACT: Australian Early Childhood Association.

Waters, J. (1996). *Making the connection: Parents and early childhood staff.* Melbourne: Lady Gowrie Child Care Centre (Melbourne) Inc.

For collaboration over issues relating to children's disabilities, you might consult:

Porter, L. & McKenzie, S. (2000). *Professional collaboration with parents of children with disabilities.* Sydney: MacLennan and Petty/London: Whurr.

17

●●

Formulating a policy

> *Busy people typically do not engage in reflection. They rarely treat themselves to reflective experiences, unless they are given some time, some structure, and the expectations to do so . . . Through reflection, we develop context-specific theories that further our own understanding of our work and generate knowledge to inform future practice.*
>
> KILLION AND TODNEM (1991: 14)

In general, policies are statements about what services you will offer and how you will deliver them. Formulating a discipline policy calls on the whole staff team, parent group and, perhaps, outside consultants to reflect on disciplinary practices. This involves active, persistent and rigorous assessment of these practices in light of the values and theory that guide them and considering their outcomes (Canning 1991).

Depending on your location, local regulations might require you to formulate policies on a range of issues, including disciplinary practices. But even where you are not required officially to document such a policy, doing so has many advantages.

Benefits of formal policies

Written policies potentially have many positive outcomes for caregivers, parents and children.

- Their procedures can guide action when a difference of opinion occurs among or between staff, families and management (Farmer 1995).
- Policies offer children, staff and parents safeguards and clear expectations of their roles, rights, and responsibilities.
- Written guidelines help to ensure that decisions about practice are consistent across time and fair to all stakeholders (Farmer 1995).
- The process of formulation is an opportunity to involve parents and staff collaboratively (Stonehouse 1991b).
- Policy development allows staff to plan in advance how to act, rather than having to make hasty decisions in response to a problem that has already occurred.
- Written documentation helps with familiarising new staff and parents with the philosophy and workings of the centre.
- Written policies assist with evaluation and accountability (Farmer 1995; Stonehouse 1991b).
- When you formulate your discipline and other policies in consultation with parents, your parent group will have a better understanding of and increased confidence in your procedures. As a result, you can be more confident that you will receive parents' support for your practices.

By far the most important advantage, however, comes not from the outcomes of policy-writing but from the process. The development of a policy gives staff and parents the opportunity to clarify their views (Stonehouse 1991b). This means that you cannot simply import the policy statement of another centre, as it is the process of clarifying what assumptions underlie practices and how the practices are intended to be enacted that gives a policy its power.

Components of a policy

Your discipline policy could comprise the following aspects (Farmer 1995): your mandate; philosophy; goals; a theoretical rationale; and a set of procedures for preventing and responding to disruptions.

Mandate

Your centre's policy needs to be framed within outside guidelines such as the code of ethical conduct for early childhood professionals (see AECA 1991; NAEYC 1989) and, for Australia, the Quality Improvement and Accreditation Guidelines (NCAC 1993). In addition, your funding body might have its own sets of policies that your centre is expected to observe.

Nevertheless, most general policies at these levels offer broad guidelines only, frequently leaving day-to-day decisions about implementation to individual centres. This is as it should be, as educators are more effective when they can exercise some discretion (Lewis 1997).

Philosophy

Many policy documents express a philosophy about behaviour management that fits within a guidance model and yet detail procedures that come from the authoritarian or controlling approaches (Lewis 1997; Porter 1999b). Discussing as a team what you believe about the philosophical debates introduced in Chapter 2 can help ensure that instead your espoused practices (detailed in subsequent sections) are consistent with your philosophy of education and of life (Edwards 2000). Specifically, you will need to answer the following questions.

- **Where do you locate children's control?** If you believe children are controlled internally, that will imply that your practices should adhere to a guidance approach; if you believe that children can and should be controlled externally, this will imply a controlling approach with its use of rewards and punishments.
- **What do you assume causes disruptive behaviour?** As a staff team, what do you think of the view espoused in this book that much of the disruptive behaviour displayed by young children is a reaction against external controls? What does your view on this issue imply for practice?
- **What is your view of children and of their mistakes**? Is this view different for developmental versus behavioural mistakes? If so, is that justified, and what does it imply for practice?

Goals

There are three levels of goals to be considered in this section: personal goals of staff; educational goals for the wider program; and goals for discipline that must be consistent with the first two.

- **Personal goals for staff**. These take account of your own personal needs and might include your requirements for a pleasant physical environment in which to work; collegial support; a measure of order in the room; courteous behaviour between all adults and children; job satisfaction; and the support of parents and centre management.
- **Educational goals.** You might highlight the goals to foster a safe and supportive environment for children (and their parents); provide an

individually relevant educational program across all domains; meet the social and emotional needs of children; encourage children to be positively disposed towards learning, and so on.

- **Disciplinary goals.** Within this wider framework, you will need to enunciate your disciplinary goals, checking as you do so that these are congruent with your educational goals. My disciplinary goals—as expressed throughout this book—comprise developing in children autonomous ethics, appropriate regulation of feelings, cooperation with others, and a sense of potency. In contrast, controlling approaches tend to emphasise compliance.

Theory

This section will describe your theoretical base. Although I have not detailed theory extensively in this book, you have read here about the differences between the controlling and guidance approaches to discipline. You could select one of these two styles or read more widely to select a theory base that is consistent with your views about education and child development, and espouses methods that are known to be ethical and effective—on all the dimensions listed in Chapter 1. (For a review of other theories, see Porter 2000a, 2000b.)

Practices

The final part of your policy document will describe what practices are to be used and by whom. Procedures will focus on how the centre can be organised so that most behavioural difficulties are prevented and those that do occur receive a constructive response (Cowin et al. 1990). These practices must conform to the ethical and philosophical stance contained in earlier sections of your policy document.

Your procedures will address:

- prevention of behavioural difficulties;
- intervention with disruptions, both those that are one-off events and those that present as chronic difficulties;
- how to facilitate parent collaboration;
- how to refer children and families to other agencies so that they receive appropriate and timely assistance from specialists when required;
- how to respond to special issues that could affect children's behaviour in the centre—such as child abuse;
- how to introduce new and relieving staff to the policy; and
- how and when to review the policy.

When roles are clearly spelled out and procedures are explicit, communication between staff is enhanced and individual staff members can feel confident about what is expected of them (Clyde 1988; Greenman & Stonehouse 1997). Therefore, it can be wise to avoid vague recommendations such as that staff will use 'positive measures' in response to disruptive behaviour, as 'positive' measures can mean different things to different people, so the actual responses involved will need to be spelled out.

Evaluation of the policy

Having worked within the policy guidelines for a specified time period, you might review its usefulness by asking yourselves the following questions (adapted from Borland 1997; Cowin et al. 1990; Davis & Rimm 1998; Sharp & Thompson 1994).

- Is your discipline plan consistent with the centre's philosophy, values, and espoused theory and with the regulations of licensing and regulatory authorities?
- Are your recommended practices realistic?
- Are the procedures being enacted as originally conceived? Do your recommendations reflect actual practice or are they a 'wish list' (Eyre 1997)?
- Are the practices achieving what you set out to accomplish?
- Are there other, important, unanticipated outcomes?
- Are there children for whom the procedures are more or less successful than others?
- If procedures need adjusting, are staff willing to carry out new approaches?
- What additional resources (including the likes of training and increased staff numbers) are necessary to make the policy more effective? Are these available?
- Are the practices an efficient use of inputs—such as the resources being used, the amount of caregivers' time, and the involvement of parents (Davis & Rimm 1998)?

You will need to review your policy regularly so that it remains relevant to workers and parents, reflects what is actually happening in the centre, and represents the best ideas and practices currently available. Although such an evaluation can seem burdensome, it can be professionally fulfilling to be able to demonstrate to yourself—if to no one else—that what you are doing is effective. Reflecting in this way on your practice can only enhance your confidence in what you do.

Conclusion

Behaviour management is most effective if everyone in the centre agrees on the values and goals that underlie practices. This can be promoted if a policy is arrived at through wide consultation. Although formulating policy by this method is time-consuming, the process gives all participants the opportunity to clarify their views and to become clear about how to enact the specified procedures.

Suggested further reading

Farmer, S. (1995). *Policy development in early childhood services*. Sydney, NSW: Community Child Care Cooperative Ltd.

Bibliography

a'Beckett, C. (1988). Parent/staff relationships. In A. Stonehouse (Ed.) *Trusting toddlers: Programming for one to three year olds in child care centres.* (pp. 140–153.) Watson, ACT: Australian Early Childhood Association.

Abbott, C.F. & Gold, S. (1991). Conferring with parents when you're concerned that their child needs special services. *Young Children, 46* (4), 10–14.

Abbott-Shim, M.S. (1990). In-service training: A means to quality care. *Young Children, 45* (2), 14–18.

Aber, J.L. & Ellwood, D.T. (2001). Thinking about children in time. In B. Bradbury, S.P. Jenkins and J. Micklewright (Eds.) *The dynamics of poverty in industrialised countries.* (pp. 281–300). Cambridge, UK: Cambridge University Press.

Adams, C. & Fay, J. (1992). *Helping your child recover from sexual abuse.* Seattle, WA: University of Washington Press.

Adler, R.B., Rosenfeld, L.B. & Proctor, R.F. II (2001). *Interplay: The process of interpersonal communication.* (8th ed.) Fort Worth, TX: Harcourt College.

Alberto P.A. & Troutman, A.C. (1999). *Applied behavior analysis for teachers.* (5th ed.) Upper Saddle River, NJ: Merrill.

Alger, H.A. (1984). Transitions: Alternatives to manipulative management techniques. *Young Children, 39* (6), 16–25.

Allen, K.E. & Schwartz, I.S. (2001). *The exceptional child: Inclusion in early childhood education.* (4th ed.) Albany, NY: Delmar.

Amatea, E.S. (1989). *Brief strategic interventions for school behavior problems.* San Francisco, CA: Jossey Bass.

Anastopoulos, A.D. & Barkley, R.A. (1992). Attention deficit-hyperactivity disorder. In C.E. Walker and M.C. Roberts (Eds.) *Handbook of clinical child psychology.* (2nd ed.) (pp. 413–430.) New York: John Wiley and Sons.

Arnett, J. (1989). Caregivers in day care centres: Does training matter? *Journal of Applied Developmental Psychology, 10*, 541–552

Arnold, D.H., Homrok, S., Ortiz, C. & Stowe, R.M. (1999). Direct observation of peer rejection acts and their temporal relation with aggressive acts. *Early Childhood Research Quarterly, 14* (2), 183–196.

Arnold, L.E. (1996), Sex differences in ADHD: Conference summary, *Journal of Abnormal Child Psychology, 24* (5), 555–569.

Arthur, L., Beecher, B., Dockett, S., Farmer, S., & Richards, E. (1996). *Programming and planning in early childhood settings.* (2nd ed.) Sydney: Harcourt Brace.

Asher, S.R. (1983). Social competence and peer status: Recent advances and future directions. *Child Development, 54,* 1427–1434.

Atwater, J.B. & Morris, E.K. (1988). Teachers' instructions and children's compliance in preschool classrooms: A descriptive analysis. *Journal of Applied Behavior Analysis, 21* (2), 157–167.

Australian Early Childhood Association (1991). Australian Early Childhood Association code of ethics. *Australian Journal of Early Childhood, 16* (1), 3–6.

Bailey, D.B. Jr (1987). Collaborative goal-setting with families: Resolving differences in values and priorities for services. *Topics in Early Childhood Special Education, 7* (2), 59–71.

Barkley, R.A. (1988). Attention deficit disorder with hyperactivity. In E.J. Mash and L.G. Terdal (Eds.) *Behavioral assessment of childhood disorders.* (2nd ed.) (pp. 69–104.) New York: Guilford.

Bass, E. & Davis, L. (1993). *Beginning to heal: A first guide for female survivors of child sexual abuse.* London: Vermilion.

Batshaw, M.L. & Conlon, C.J. (1997). Substance abuse: A preventable threat to development. In M.L. Batshaw (Ed.) *Children with disabilities.* (4th ed.) (pp. 143–162.) Sydney: MacLennan & Petty.

Boyd, H. (1998). *The step-parent's survival guide.* London: Ward Lock.

Baumrind, D. (1967). Child care practices anteceding three patterns of preschool behavior. *Genetic Psychology Monographs, 75,* 43–88.

(1971). Current patterns of parental authority. *Developmental Psychology Monograph, 4* (1), 1–103.

Bay-Hinitz, A.K., Peterson, R.F. & Quilitch, R. (1994). Cooperative games: A way to modify aggressive and cooperative behaviors in young children. *Journal of Applied Behavior Analysis, 27* (3), 435–446.

Bentley-Williams, R. & Butterfield, N. (1996). Transition from early intervention to school: A family focussed view of the issues involved. *Australasian Journal of Special Education, 20* (2), 17–28.

Bergen, D. (1994). Should teachers permit or discourage violent play themes? *Childhood Education, 70* (5), 300–301.

Berne, P.H. & Savary, L.M. (1996). *Building self-esteem in children.* (exp. ed.) New York: Crossroad Publishing.

Bevill, A.R. & Gast, D.L. (1998). Social safety for young children: A review of the literature on safety skills instruction. *Topics in Early Childhood Special Education, 18* (4), 222–234.

Biddulph, S. (1993). *The secret of happy children.* (rev. ed.) Sydney: Bay Books.

Billman, J. (1995). Child care program directors: What skills do they need? Results of a statewide survey. *Early Childhood Education Journal, 23* (2), 63–70.

Birch, L.L., Johnson, S.L. & Fischer, J.A. (1995). Children's eating: The development of food-acceptance patterns. *Young Children, 50* (2), 71–78.

—— (1999). Children's eating: The development of food-acceptance patterns. In L. Berk (Ed.) Landscapes of development: An anthology of readings. (pp. 195–206.) Belmont, CA: Wadsworth.

Bloom, P.J. (1982). *Avoiding burnout: Strategies for managing time, space, and people in early childhood education*. Lake Forest, IL: New Horizons.

Blum, N.J. & Mercugliano, M. (1997). Attention-deficit/hyperactivity disorder. In M.L. Batshaw (Ed.) *Children with disabilities*. (4th ed.) (pp. 449–470.) Sydney: MacLennan and Petty.

Bolton, R. (1987). *People skills*. Sydney: Simon and Schuster.

Bonner, B.L., Kaufman, K.L., Harbeck, C. & Brassard, M.R. (1992). Child maltreatment. In C.E. Walker and M.C. Roberts (Eds.) *Handbook of clinical child psychology*. (2nd ed.) (pp. 967–1008.) New York: John Wiley and Sons.

Booth, T. & Booth, W. (1995). Unto us a child is born: The trials and rewards of parenthood for people with learning difficulties. *Australia and New Zealand Journal of Developmental Disabilities*, 20 (1), 25–39.

Borland, J.H. (1997). Evaluating gifted programs. In N. Colangelo and G.A. Davis (Eds.) *Handbook of gifted education*. (2nd ed.) (pp. 253–266.) Boston, MA: Allyn and Bacon.

Bouchard, L.L. (1991). Mixed age groupings for gifted students. *Gifted Child Today*, 14 (5), 30–35.

Boutte, G.S., Keepler, D.L., Tyler, V.S. & Terry, B.Z. (1992). Effective techniques for involving 'difficult' parents. *Young Children*, 47 (3), 19–22.

Bowman, B.T. & Stott, F.M. (1994). Understanding development in a cultural context. In B.L. Mallory and R.S. New (Eds.) *Diversity and developmental appropriate practices: Challenges for early childhood education*. (pp. 119–133.) New York: Teachers College Press.

Boyd, H. (1998). *The step-parent's survival guide*. London: Ward Lock.

Bradbury, B., Jenkins, S.P. & Micklewright, J. (2001). Beyond the snapshot: A dynamic view of child poverty. In B. Bradbury, S.P. Jenkins and J. Micklewright (Eds.) *The dynamics of poverty in industrialised countries*. (pp. 1–23). Cambridge, UK: Cambridge University Press.

Brand, S.F. (1990). Undergraduates and beginning preschool teachers working with young children: Educational and developmental issues. *Young Children*, 45 (2), 19–24.

Bredekamp, S. & Copple, C. (Eds.) (1997). *Developmentally appropriate practice in early childhood programs*. (rev. ed.) Washington, DC: National Association for the Education of Young Children.

Briggs, F. (1993). *Why my child? Supporting the families of victims of child sexual abuse*. Sydney: Allen and Unwin.

Briggs, F. & McVeity, M. (2000). *Teaching children to protect themselves*. Sydney: Allen and Unwin.

Brinegar, J. (1992). *Breaking free from domestic violence*. Center City, MN: CompCare Publishers.

Broinowski, I. (1994). *Managing child care centres*. Melbourne, Vic: TAFE Publications.

Brown, P.M., Remine, M.D., Prescott, S.J. & Rickards, F.W. (2000). Social interactions of preschoolers with and without impaired hearing in integrated kindergarten. *Journal of Early Intervention*, 23 (3), 200–211.

Buchanan, T. & Burts, D. (1995). Getting parents involved in the 1990s. *Day Care and Early Education, 22* (4), 18–22.

Burns, A. & Goodnow, J. (1985). *Children and families in Australia.* (2nd ed.) Sydney: Allen and Unwin.

Burns, R.B. (1982). *Self-concept development and education.* London: Holt, Rhinehart and Winston.

Burrett, J. (1999). *But I want to stay with you: Talking with children about separation and divorce.* Sydney: Simon and Schuster.

Buysse, V., Wesley, P.W. & Keyes, L. (1998). Implementing early childhood inclusion: Barrier and support factors. *Early Childhood Research Quarterly, 13* (1), 169–184.

Canning, C. (1991). What teachers say about reflection. *Educational Leadership, 48* (6), 18–21.

Caruso, J.J. (1991). Supervisors in early childhood programs: An emerging profile. *Young Children, 46* (6), 20–26.

Caughey, C. (1991). Becoming the child's ally—observations in a classroom for children who have been abused. *Young Children, 46* (4), 22–28.

Chandler, P.A. (1994). *A place for me: Including children with special needs in early care and education settings.* Washington, DC: National Association for the Education of Young Children.

Clark, B. (1997). *Growing up gifted: Developing the potential of children at home and at school.* (5th ed.) Upper Saddle River, NJ: Merrill.

Clyde, M. (1988). Staff burnout—the ultimate reward? In A. Stonehouse (Ed.) *Trusting toddlers: Programming for one to three year olds in child care centres.* (pp. 170–177.) Watson, ACT: Australian Early Childhood Association.
(1995). Concluding the debate: Mind games—what DAP means to me. In M. Fleer (Ed.) *DAPcentrism: Challenging developmentally appropriate practice.* (pp. 109–116.) Watson, ACT: Australian Early Childhood Association.

Cohn, J.F. & Campbell, S.B. (1992). Influence of maternal depression on infant affect regulation. In D. Cicchetti & S.L. Toth (Eds.) *Developmental perspectives on depression: Rochester symposium on developmental psychopathology.* (vol. 4) (pp. 103–130.) Rochester, NY: University of Rochester Press.

Cole-Detke, H. & Kobak, R. (1998). The effects of multiple abuse in interpersonal relationships: An attachment perspective. In B.B.R. Rossman & M.S. Rosenberg (Eds.) *Multiple victimization of children: Conceptual, developmental, research and treatment isssues.* (pp. 189–205.) New York: Haworth Press.

Conlon, A. (1992). Giving Mrs Jones a hand: Making group storytime more pleasurable and meaningful for young children. *Young Children, 47* (3), 14–18

Conway, R. (1998). Meeting the needs of students with behavioural and emotional problems. In A. Ashman and J. Elkins (Eds.) *Educating children with special needs.* (3rd ed.) (pp. 177–228.) Sydney: Prentice Hall.

Coopersmith, S. (1967). *The antecedents of self-esteem.* San Francisco, CA: W.H. Freeman.

Cornell, D.G., Delcourt, M.A.B., Bland, L.C., Goldberg, M.D. & Oram, G. (1994). Low incidence of behavior problems among elementary school students in gifted programs. *Journal for the Education of the Gifted, 18* (1), 4–19.

Covaleskie, J.F. (1992). Discipline and morality: Beyond rules and consequences. *The Educational Forum, 56* (2), 173–183.

Cowin, M., Freeman, L., Farmer, A., James, M., Drent, A. & Arthur, R. (1990). *Positive school discipline: A practical guide to developing policy.* (rev. ed.) Boronia, Vic: Narbethong Publications.

Crary, E. (1992). Talking about differences children notice. In B. Neugebauer (Ed.) *Alike and different: Exploring our humanity with young children.* (rev. ed.) (pp. 11–15.) Washington, DC: National Association for the Education of Young Children.

Crockenberg, S. & Litman, C. (1990). Autonomy as competence in 2-year-olds: Maternal correlates of child defiance, compliance, and self-assertion. *Developmental Psychology, 26* (6), 961–971.

Cummings, E.M. (1998). Stress and coping approaches and research: The impact of marital conflict on children. In B.B.R. Rossman and M.S. Rosenberg (Eds.) *Multiple victimization of children: Conceptual, developmental, research, and treatment issues.* (pp. 31–50). New York: Haworth Press.

Cupit, C.G. (1989). *Socialising the superheroes.* Watson, ACT: Australian Early Childhood Association.

Curry, N.E. & Johnson, C.N. (1990). *Beyond self-esteem: Developing a genuine sense of human value.* Washington, DC: National Association for the Education of Young Children.

Dahlberg, G., Moss, P. & Pence, A. (1999). *Beyond quality in early childhood education and care: Postmodern perspectives.* London: Routledge Falmer.

Dau, E. (2001). *The anti-bias approach in early childhood.* (2nd ed.) Sydney: Addison-Wesley.

David, T. (1999). Valuing young children. In L. Abbott and H. Moylett (Eds.) *Early education transformed.* (pp. 82–92.) London: Falmer.

Davis, L. (1991). *Allies in healing: When the person you love was sexually abused as a child.* New York: Harper Perennial.

Davis, G.A. & Rimm, S.B. (1998). *Education of the gifted and talented.* (4th ed.) Boston, MA: Allyn and Bacon.

Dawkins, M. (1991). Hey dudes, what's the rap?: A plea for leniency towards superhero play. *Australian Journal of Early Childhood, 16* (2), 3–8.

de Shazer, S. (1993). Creative misunderstanding: There is no escape from language. In S. Gilligan and R. Price (Eds.) *Therapeutic conversations.* (pp. 81–135.) New York: W.W. Norton.

de Shazer, S., Berg, I.K., Lipchik, E., Nunnally, E., Molnar, A., Gingerich, W. & Weiner-Davis, M. (1986). Brief therapy: Focused solution development. *Family Process, 25* (2), 207–222.

Dengate, S. (1997). Dietary management of attention deficit disorder. *Australian Journal of Early Childhood, 22* (4), 29–33.

Derman-Sparks, L. (1992). 'It isn't fair!' Antibias curriculum for young children. In B. Neugebauer (Ed.) *Alike and different: Exploring our humanity with young children*. (rev. ed.) (pp. 2–10.) Washington, DC: National Association for the Education of Young Children.

Derman-Sparks, L. & the A.B.C. Task Force (1989). *Anti-bias curriculum: Tools for empowering young children*. Washington, DC: National Association for the Education of Young Children.

Dinnebeil, L.A., McInerney, W., Fox, C. & Juchartz-Pendry, K. (1998). An analysis of the perceptions and characteristics of childcare personnel regarding inclusion of young children with special needs in community-based programs. *Topics in Early Childhood Special Education, 18* (2), 118–128.

Dodge, K.A. (1983). Behavioral antecedents of peer social status. *Child Development, 54,* 1386–1399.

Doherty-Derkowski, G. (1995). *Quality matters: Excellence in early childhood programs*. Don Mills, Ontario: Addison-Wesley.

Doyle, W. (1986). Classroom organization and management. In M.C. Wittrock (Ed.) *Handbook of research on teaching*. (3rd ed.) (pp. 392–431.) New York: Macmillan.

Durrant, M. (1995). *Creative strategies for school problems*. Epping, NSW: Eastwood Family Therapy Centre/New York: Norton.

Edwards, C.H. (2000). *Classroom discipline and management*. (3rd ed.) New York: Wiley.

Elicker, J. & Fortner-Wood, C. (1995). Adult-child relationships in early childhood programs. *Young Children, 51* (1), 69–78.

Evans, P. (1996). *The verbally abusive relationship: How to recognize it and how to respond*. (exp. 2nd ed.) Holbrook, MA: Adams Media Corporation.

Eyre, D. (1997). *Able children in ordinary schools*. London: David Fulton.

Faber, A., Mazlish, E., Nyberg, L. & Templeton, R.A. (1995). *How to talk so kids can learn at home and in school*. New York: Fireside.

Faber, A. & Mazlish, E. (1999). *How to talk so kids will listen and listen so kids will talk*. New York: Avon.

Farmer, S. (1995). *Policy development in early childhood services*. Newtown, NSW: Community Child Care Cooperative Ltd.

Farver, J.M. (1996). Aggressive behavior in preschoolers' social networks: Do birds of a feather flock together? *Early Childhood Research Quarterly, 11* (3), 333–350.

Feldman, M.A. (1994). Parenting education for parents with intellectual disabilities: A review of outcome studies. *Research in Developmental Disabilities, 15* (4), 299–332.

Feldman, M.A., Case, L., Rincover, A., Towns, F. & Betel, J. (1989). Parent education project III: Increasing affection and responsivity in developmentally handicapped mothers: Component analysis, generalization, and effects on child language. *Journal of Applied Behavior Analysis, 22* (2), 211–222.

Feldhusen, J.F. (1989). Synthesis of research on gifted youths. *Educational Leadership*, 46 (6), 6–11.

Field, T. (1989). Maternal depression effects on infant interaction and attachment behavior. In D. Cicchetti (Ed.) *The emergence of a discipline: Rochester symposium on developmental psychopathology.* (vol. 1) (pp. 139–163). Hillsdale, NJ: Lawrence Erlbaum.

—— (1992). Infants of depressed mothers. Development and Psychopathology, 4 (1), 49–66.

Field, T., Vega-Lahr, N., Scafidi, F. & Goldstein, S. (1986). Effects of infant unavailability on mother-infant interactions. *Infant Behavior and Development*, 9 (4), 473–478.

Fields, M. & Boesser, C. (2002). *Constructive guidance and discipline.* (3rd ed.) Upper Saddle River, NJ: Merrill Prentice Hall.

Fisch, R., Weakland, J.H. & Segal, L. (1982). *The tactics of change: Doing therapy briefly.* San Francisco, CA: Jossey-Bass.

Fitzgerald, H. (1992). *The grieving child: A parent's guide.* New York: Fireside.

Fleet, A. & Clyde, M. (1993). *What's in a day? Working in early childhood.* Wentworth Falls, NSW: Social Science Press.

Fowler, S.A., Schwartz, I. & Atwater, J. (1991). Perspectives on the transition from preschool to kindergarten for children with disabilities and their families. *Exceptional Children*, 58 (2), 136–145.

Fox, A.M. & Rieder, M.J. (1993). Risks and benefits of drugs used in the management of the hyperactive child. *Drug Safety*, 9 (1), 38–50.

Fraser, S. & Gestwicki, C. (2002). *Authentic childhood: Exploring Reggio Emilia in the classroom.* Albany, NY: Delmar.

Freeman, S.F.N. & Kasari, C. (1998). Friendships in children with developmental disabilities. *Early Education and Development*, 9 (4), 341–355.

Galinsky, E. (1988). Parents and teacher-caregivers: Sources of tension, sources of support. *Young Children*, 43 (3), 4–12.

—— (1989). A parent/teacher study: Interesting results. *Young Children*, 45 (1), 2–3.

—— (1990). Why are some parent/teacher partnerships clouded with difficulties? *Young Children*, 45 (5), 2–3; 38–9.

Gallucci, N.T. (1988). Emotional adjustment of gifted children. *Gifted Child Quarterly*, 32 (2), 273–276.

Gartrell, D. (1987). Punishment or guidance? *Young Children*, 42 (3), 55–61.

(1998). *A guidance approach for the encouraging classroom.* New York: Delmar.

George, C. & Main, M. (1979). Social interactions of young abused children: Approach, avoidance, and aggression. *Child Development*, 50 (2), 306–318.

Gerber, M. (1981). What is appropriate curriculum for infants and toddlers?. In B. Weissbourd and J. Musick (Eds.) *Infants: Their social environments.* (pp. 77–85.) Washington, DC: National Association fo the Education of Young Children.

Gestwicki, C. (1995). *Developmentally appropriate practice: Curriculum development in early education.* Albany, NY: Delmar.

Gilding, M. (1997). *Australian families: A comparative perspective*. South Melbourne: Longman.

Ginott, H. (1972). *Teacher and child*. New York: Macmillan.

Glasser, W. (1998). *The quality school: Managing students without coercion*. (rev. ed.) New York: Harper Perennial.

Goldstein, M. & Goldstein, S. (1995). Medications and behavior in the classroom. In S. Goldstein (Ed.) *Understanding and managing children's classroom behavior*. (pp. 181–219.) New York: John Wiley and Sons.

Goldstein, S. (1995). Attention deficit hyperactivity disorder. In S. Goldstein (Ed.) *Understanding and managing children's classroom behavior*. (pp. 56–78.) New York: John Wiley and Sons.

Goodman, S.H. & Brumley, H.E. (1990). Schizophrenic and depressed mothers: Relational deficits in parenting. *Developmental Psychology, 26* (1), 31–39.

Goodnow, J.J. (1989). Setting priorities for research on group care of children. *Australian Journal of Early Childhood, 14* (1), 4–10.

Gootman, M.E. (1993). Reaching and teaching abused children. *Childhood Education, 70* (1), 15–19.

Gordon, T. (1970). *Parent effectiveness training*. New York: Plume.

—— (1974). *Teacher effectiveness training*. New York: Peter H. Wyden.

—— (1991). *Teaching children self-discipline at home and at school*. Sydney: Random House.

Gowen, J.W. & Nebrig, J.B. (2002). *Enhancing early emotional development: Guiding parents of young children*. Baltimore, MD: Paul H. Brookes.

Grant, G., Ramcharan, P., McGrath, M., Nolan, M. & Keady, J. (1998). Rewards and gratifications among family caregivers. *Journal of Intellectual Disability Research, 42* (1), 58–71.

Graue, M.E. & Walsh, D.J. (1998). *Studying children in context: Theories, methods and ethics*. Thousand Oaks, CA: SAGE.

Green, C. & Chee, K. (1997). *Understanding ADHD: A parent's guide to attention-deficit hyperactivity disorder in children*. Sydney: Random House.

Greenberg, P. (1992). Ideas that work with young children: How to institute some simple democratic practices pertaining to respect, rights, roots and responsibilities in any classroom (without losing your leadership position). *Young Children, 47* (5), 10–17.

Greenman, J. & Stonehouse, A. (1997). *Prime times: A handbook for excellence in infant and toddler programs*. South Melbourne: Longman.

Gronlund, G. (1992). Coping with Ninja turtle play in my kindergarten classroom. *Young Children, 48* (1), 21–25.

Guralnick, M.J. (1991). The next decade of research on the effectiveness of early intervention. *Exceptional Children, 58* (2), 174–183.

Guralnick, M.J., Connor, R.T., Hammond, M., Gottman, J.M. & Kinnish, K. (1995). Immediate effects of mainstreamed settings on the social interactions and social integration of preschool children. *American Journal on Mental Retardation, 100* (4), 359–377.

Guralnick, M.J., Paul-Brown, D., Groom, J.M., Booth, C.L., Hammond, M.A., Tupper, D.B. & Gelenter, A. (1998). Conflict resolution patterns of preschool children with and without developmental delays in heterogeneous playgroups. *Early Education and Development, 9* (1), 49–77.

Hanson, M.J. & Carta, J.J. (1995). Addressing the challenges of families with multiple risks. *Exceptional Children, 62* (3), 201–212.

Harrison, C. (1999). *Giftedness in early childhood.* (2nd ed.) Sydney: Gerric.

Harrison, C. & Tegel, K. (1999). Play and the gifted child. In E. Dau (Ed.) *Child's play: Revisiting play in early childhood settings.* (pp. 97–110.) Sydney: MacLennan and Petty.

Hart-Byers, S. (1998). *Secrets of successful step-families.* Port Melbourne: Lothian.

Harter, S. (1998). The effects of child abuse on the self-esteem. In B.B.R. Rossman & M.S. Rosenberg (Eds.) *Multiple victimization of children: Conceptual, developmental, research and treatment issues.* (pp. 147–169.) New York: Haworth Press.

Hartup, W.W. (1989). Social relationships and their developmental significance. *American Psychologist, 44* (2), 120–126.

Hartup, W.W. & Moore, S.G. (1990). Early peer relations: Developmental significance and prognostic implications. *Early Childhood Research Quarterly, 5* (1), 1–17.

Hauser-Cram, P., Bronson, M.B. & Upshur, C.C. (1993). The effects of classroom environment on the social and mastery behavior of preschool children with disabilities. *Early Childhood Research Quarterly, 8* (4), 479–497.

Heath, H.E. (1994). Dealing with difficult behaviors: Teachers plan with parents. *Young Children, 49* (5), 20–24.

Herbert, M. (1987). *Behavioural treatment of children with problems: A practice manual.* (2nd ed.) London: Academic Press.

Hill, S. & Reed, K. (1989). Promoting social competence at preschool: The implementation of a cooperative games programme. *Australian Journal of Early Childhood, 14* (4), 25–31.

Hilliard, A.G. (1985). What is quality care? In B.M. Caldwell and A.G. Hilliard III (Eds.) *What is quality care?* (pp. 17–32.) Washington, DC: National Association for the Education of Young Children.

Hinshaw, S.P. (2000). Attention-deficit/hyperactivity disorder: The search of viable treatments. In P.C. Kendall (Ed.) *Child and adolescent therapy: Cognitive-behavioral procedures.* (2nd ed.) (pp. 88–128.) New York: Guilford.

Hoffman-Plotkin, D. & Twentyman, C.T. (1984). A multimodal assessment of behavioral and cognitive deficits in abused and neglected preschoolers. *Child Development, 55* (3), 794–802.

Howard, V.F., Williams, B.F., Port, P.D. & Lepper, C. (2001). *Very young children with special needs: A formative approach for the 21st century.* (2nd ed.) Upper Saddle River, NJ: Merrill Prentice Hall.

Howes, C. (1983a). Patterns of friendship. *Child Development, 54* (4), 1041–1053. (1983b). Caregiver behavior in center and family day care. *Journal of Applied Developmental Psychology, 4,* 99–107.

Hunter, M. (1990). *Abused boys: The neglected victims of sexual abuse.* New York: Fawcett Columbine.

Ivory, J.J. & McCollum J.A. (1999). Effects of social and isolate toys on social play in an inclusive setting. *The Journal of Special Education, 32* (4), 238–243.

Jakubowski, P. & Lange, A. J. (1978). *The assertive option: Your rights and responsibilities.* Champaign, IL: Research Press.

Jones, V.F. & Jones, L.S. (2001). *Comprehensive classroom management: Creating communities of support and solving problems.* (6th ed.) Boston, MA: Allyn and Bacon.

Jordan, N.H. (1993). Sexual abuse prevention programs in early childhood education: A caveat. *Young Children, 48* (6), 76–79.

Jorde-Bloom, P. (1988). Teachers need 'TLC' too. *Young Children, 43* (6), 4–8.

Kamii, C. (1985). Autonomy: The aim of education envisioned by Piaget. *Australian Journal of Early Childhood, 10* (1), 3–10.

Kaplan, J.S. & Carter, J. (1995). *Beyond behavior modification: A cognitive-behavioral approach to behavior management in the school.* (3rd ed.) Austin, TX: Pro-Ed.

Katsurada, E. & Sugawara, A.I. (1998). The relationship between hostile attributional bias and aggressive behavior in preschoolers. *Early Childhood Research Quarterly, 13* (4), 623–636.

Katz, L.G. (1995). *Talks with teachers of young children.* Norwood, NJ: Ablex.

Katz, L.G., Evangelou, D. & Hartman, J.A. (1990). *The case for mixed-age grouping in early education.* Washington, DC: National Association for the Education of Young Children.

Katz, L.G. & McClellan, D.E. (1997). *Fostering children's social competence: The teacher's role.* Washington, DC: National Association for the Education of Young Children.

Kelly, B. (1996). The ecology of peer relations. *Early Child Development and Care, 115,* 99–114.

Killion, J.P. & Todnem, G.R. (1991). A process for personal theory building. *Educational Leadership, 48* (6), 14–16.

King, H.E. (1992). The reactions of children to divorce. In C.E. Walker and M.C. Roberts (Eds.) *Handbook of clinical child psychology.* (2nd ed.) (pp. 1009–1024.) New York: Plenum.

Klass, C.S. (1999). *The child care provider: Promoting young children's development.* Baltimore, MD: Paul H. Brookes.

Kleinman, H. (1988). What are parents concerned about? In A. Godwin and L. Schrag (Eds.) *Setting up for infant care: Guidelines for centers and family day care homes.* Washington, DC: National Association for the Education of Young Children.

Klimes-Dougan, B. & Kistner, J. (1990). Physically abused preschoolers' responses to peers' distress. *Developmental Psychology, 26* (4), 599–602.

Kohn, A. (1996). *Beyond discipline: From compliance to community.* Alexandria, VA: Association for Supervision and Curriculum Development.

—— (1999). *Punished by rewards: The trouble with gold stars, incentive plans, A's, praise and other bribes.* (2nd ed.) Boston, MA: Houghton Mifflin.

Kontos, S. & Wilcox-Herzog, A. (1997). Teachers' interactions with children: Why are they so important? *Young Children, 52* (2), 4–12.

Kostelnick, M.J., Stein, L.C., Whiren, A.P. & Soderman, A.K. (1998). *Guiding children's social development.* (3rd ed.) Albany, NY: Delmar.

Kral, R. & Kowalski, K. (1989). After the miracle: The second stage in solution focused brief therapy. *Journal of Strategic and Systemic Therapies, 8* (2), 73–76.

Ladd, G.W. & Mize, J. (1983). Social skills training and assessment with children: A cognitive-social learning approach. In C.W. LeCroy (Ed.) *Social skills training for children and youth.* (pp. 61–74.) New York: Haworth Press.

Lady Gowrie Child Centre Melbourne Inc. (1987). *Aspects of quality day care: An evaluative summary of recent literature.* North Carlton, VIC: author.

Lambert, B. (1994). *Beating burnout: A multi-dimensional perspective.* AECA Resource Book Series, 1 (2). Watson, ACT: Australian Early Childhood Association.

Lambert, E.B. & Clyde, M. (2000). *Re-thinking early childhood theory and practice.* Katoomba, NSW: Social Science Press.

Larner, M. & Phillips, D. (1994). Defining and valuing quality as a parent. In P. Moss and A. Pence (Eds.) *Transforming nursery education.* (pp. 43–60.) London: Paul Chapman.

Levy, F. (1993). Side effects of stimulant use. *Journal of Paediatric Child Health, 29,* 250–254.

Lew, M. (1990). *Victims no longer: A guide for men recovering from sexual child abuse.* London: Cedar.

Lewis, R. (1997). *The discipline dilemma.* (2nd ed.) Melbourne: A.C.E.R.

Lieber, J., Capell, K., Sandall, S.R., Wolfberg, P., Horn, e. & Beckman, P. (1998). Inclusive prescholl programs; Teachers' beliefs and practices. *Early Childhood Research Quarterly,* 13 (1), 87–105.

Llewellyn, G. (1990). People with intellectual disability as parents: Perspectives from the professional literature. *Australia and New Zealand Journal of Developmental Disabilities, 16* (4), 369–380.

—— (1994). Generic family support services: Are parents with learning disability catered for? *Mental Handicap Research, 7* (1), 64–77.

—— (1995). Relationships and social support: Views of parents with mental retardation/intellectual disability. *Mental Retardation, 33* (6), 349–363.

Llewellyn, G. & Brigden, D. (1995). Factors affecting service provision to parents with intellectual disability: An exploratory study. *Australia and New Zealand Journal of Developmental Disabilities, 20* (2), 97–112.

Llewellyn, G., Thompson, K. & Proctor, A. (1999). Early intervention services and parents with disabilities. *International Journal of Practical Approaches to Disability, 23* (1), 3–8.

Lloyd, L. (1997). Multi-age classes: An option for all students? *The Australasian Journal of Gifted Education, 6* (1), 46–54.

Luthar, S.S. & Zigler, E. (1991). Vulnerability and competence: A review of the research on resilience in childhood. *American Journal of Orthopsychiatry*, 6, 6–22.

Lyons-Ruth, K. (1992). Maternal depressive symptoms, disorganized infant-mother attachment relationships and hostile-aggressive behavior in the preschool classroom: A prospective longitudinal view from infancy to age five. In D. Cicchetti & S.L. Toth (Eds.) *Developmental perspectives on depression: Rochester symposium on developmental psychopathology.* (vol. 4) (pp. 131–171.) Rochester, NY: University of Rochester Press.

Lyons-Ruth, K., Zoll, D., Connell, D. & Grunebaum, H.U. (1986). The depressed mother and her one-year-old infant: Environment, interaction, attachment, and infant development. *New Directions for Child Development, 34*, 61–82.

Mackay, H. (1994). *The good listener.* Sydney: Macmillan.

MacMullin, C.E. & Napper, M. (1993). Teachers and inclusion of students with disabilities: Attitude, confidence or encouragement? Paper presented to the *Australian Early Intervention Association (SA Chapter) Conference.* Adelaide: June 1993.

MacNaughton, G. & Williams, G. (1998). *Techniques for teaching young children: Choices in theory and practice.* Sydney: Longman.

Marecek, M. (1993). *Breaking free from partner abuse: Voices of battered women caught in the cycle of domestic violence.* Buena Park, CA: Morning Glory Press.

Mason, D.A. & Burns, R.B. (1996). 'Simply no worse and simply no better' may simply be wrong: A critique of Veenman's conclusion about multigrade classes. *Review of Educational Research, 66* (3), 307–322.

McCaslin, M. & Good, T.L. (1992). Compliant cognition: The misalliance of management and instructional goals in current school reform. *Educational Researcher, 21* (3), 4–17.

McCollum, J.A. & Bair, H. (1994). Research in parent-child interaction. Guidance to developmentally appropriate practice for young children with disabilities. In B.L. Mallory and R.S. New (Eds.) *Diversity and developmental appropriate practices: Challenges for early childhood education.* (pp. 84–106.) New York: Teachers College Press.

McConnell, D., Llewellyn, G. & Bye, R. (1997). Providing services for parents with intellectual disability: Parent needs and service constraints. *Journal of Intellectual and Developmental Disability, 22* (1), 5–17.

McDonald, P. (1993). *Family trends and structure in Australia.* Melbourne: Australian Institute of Family Studies.

McDonnell, A.P., Brownell, K. & Wolery, M. (1997). Teaching experience and specialist support: A survey of preschool teachers employed in programs accredited by NAEYC. *Topics in Early Childhood Special Education, 17* (3), 263–285.

McKissock, D. (1998). *The grief of our children.* Sydney: ABC.

McKissock, M. & McKissock, D. (1995). *Coping with grief.* (3rd ed.) Sydney: ABC.

Meyer, D.J. (1993). Lessons learned: Cognitive coping strategies of overlooked family members. In A.P. Turnbull, J.M. Patterson, S.K. Behr, D.L. Murphy, J.G. Marquis and M.J. Blue-Banning (Eds.) *Cognitive coping, families and disability* (pp. 81–93.) Baltimore, MD: Paul H. Brookes.

Mitchell, G. (1993). *Help! What do I do about . . .?* New York: Scholastic.

Mize, J. (1995). Coaching preschool children in social skills: A cognitive-social learning curriculum. In G. Cartledge and J.F. Milburn (Eds.) *Teaching social skills to children and youth: Innovative approaches.* (3rd ed.) (pp. 237–261.) New York: Pergamon.

Molnar, A. & de Shazer, S. (1987). Solution-focused therapy: Toward the identification of therapeutic tasks. *Journal of Marital and Family Therapy, 13* (4), 349–358.

Molnar, A. & Lindquist, B. (1989). *Changing problem behaviour in schools.* San Francisco, CA: Jossey-Bass.

Moss, P. (1999). Early childhood institutions as a democratic and emancipatory project. In L. Abbott and H. Moylett (Eds.) *Early education transformed.* (pp. 142–152.) London: Falmer.

Mosteller, F., Light, R.J. & Sachs, J.A. (1996). Sustained inquiry in education: Lessons from skill grouping and class size. *Harvard Educational Review, 66* (4), 797–842.

Mruk, C.J. (1999). *Self-esteem: Research, theory and practice.* (2nd ed.) London: Free Association Books.

National Association for the Education of Young Children (1983). Four components of high quality early childhood programs: Staff-child interaction, child-child interaction, curriculum, and evaluation. *Young Children, 38* (6), 46–52.

—— (1984). Criteria for high quality early childhood programs. *Position paper from the National Academy of Early Childhood Programs,* 3–13.

—— (1989). Code of ethical conduct. *Young Children, 45* (1), 25–29.

National Childcare Accreditation Council (1993). *Putting children first: Quality improvement and accreditation system handbook.* Sydney: National Childcare Accreditation Council.

O'Donnell, C. & Craney, J. (1982). Incest and the reproduction of the patriarchal family. In C. O'Donnell and J. Craney (Eds.) *Family violence in Australia.* Melbourne: Longman Cheshire.

Odom, S.L., McConnell, S.R. & McEvoy, M.A. (Eds.) (1992). *Social competence of young children with disabilities: Issues and strategies for intervention.* Baltimore, MD: Paul H. Brookes.

Odom, S.L., McConnell, S.R., McEvoy, M.A., Peterson, C., Ostrosky, M., Chandler, L.K., Spicuzza, R.J., Skellenger, A., Creighton, M. & Favazza, P.C. (1999). Relative effects of interventions supporting the social competence of young children with disabilities. *Topics in Early Childhood Special Education, 19* (2), 75–91.

Okagaki, L., Diamond, K.E., Kontos, S.J. & Hestenes, L.L. (1998). Correlates of young children's interactions with classmates with disabilities. *Early Childhood Research Quarterly, 13* (1), 67–86.

Orlick, T. (1982). *The second cooperative sports and games book.* New York: Pantheon.

Parker, W. & Adkins, K.K. (1995). Perfectionism and the gifted. *Roeper Review, 17* (3), 173–176.

Parpal, M. & Maccoby, E.E. (1985). Maternal responsiveness and subsequent child compliance. *Child Development, 56* (5), 1326–1334.

Perkins, D.N., Jay, E. & Tishman, S. (1993). Beyond abilities: A dispositional theory of thinking. *Merrill Palmer Quarterly 39* (1), 1–21.

Perleth, C., Schatz, T. & Mönks, F.J. (2000). Early identification of high ability. In K.A. Heller, F.J. Mönks, R.J. Sternberg and R.F. Subotnik (Eds.) *International handbook of giftedness and talent.* (2nd ed.) (pp. 297–316.) Oxford, UK: Pergamon.

Peterson, C. (1996). *Looking forward through the life span: Developmental psychology.* (3rd ed.) Sydney: Prentice Hall.

Phillips, D.A. & Howes, C. (1987). Indicators of quality child care: Review of research. In D. Phillips (Ed.) *Quality in child care: What does research tell us?* (pp. 1–19.) Washington, DC: National Association for the Education of Young Children.

Pope, A.W., McHale, S.M., & Craighead, E.W. (1988). *Self-esteem enhancement with children and adolescents.* New York: Pergamon.

Porteous, M.A. (1979). A survey of the problems of normal 15-year-olds. *Journal of Adolescence, 2* (4), 307–323.

Porter, L. (1999a). *Gifted young children: A guide for teachers and parents.* Sydney: Allen and Unwin/ Buckingham, UK: Open University Press.

—— (1999b). *Behaviour management practices in child care centres.* Unpublished doctoral thesis. Adelaide: University of South Australia.

—— (2000a). *Student behaviour: Theory and practice for teachers.* (2nd ed.) Sydney: Allen and Unwin.

—— (2000b). *Behaviour in schools: Theory and practice for teachers.* Buckinghmam, UK: Open University Press.

—— (Ed.) (2002a.) *Educating young children with additional needs.* Sydney: Allen and Unwin.

—— (Ed.) (2002b). *Educating young children with special needs.* London: Paul Chapman/Thousand Oaks, CA: SAGE.

Porter, L. & McKenzie, S. (2000). *Professional collaboration with parents of children with disabilities.* Sydney: MacLennan and Petty/London: Whurr.

Powell, D.R. (1994). Parents, pluralism, and the NAEYC statement on developmentally appropriate practice. In B.L. Mallory and R.S. New (Eds.) *Diversity and developmental appropriate practices: Challenges for early childhood education.* (pp. 166–182.) New York: Teachers College Press.

Pugh, G. & Selleck, D.R. (1996). Listening to and communicating with young children. In R. Davie, G. Upton and V. Varma (Eds.) *The voice of the child: A handbook for professionals* (pp. 120–136.) London: Falmer Press.

Putallaz, M. & Gottman, J.M. (1981). An interactional model of children's entry into peer groups. *Child Development, 52* (3), 986–994.

Putallaz, M. & Wasserman, A. (1990). Children's entry behavior. In S.R. Asher and J.D. Coie (Eds.) *Peer rejection in childhood.* (pp. 60–89.) Cambridge, UK: Cambridge University Press.

Raban, B. (1997). What counts towards quality provision? *International Journal of Early Childhood, 29* (1), 57–63.

Ramey, C.T. & Ramey, S.L. (1992). Effective early intervention. *Mental Retardation, 30* (6), 337–345.

Readdick, C.A. (1993). Solitary pursuits: Supporting children's privacy needs in early childhood settings. *Young Children, 49* (1), 60–64.

Richarz, S. (1993). Innovations in early childhood education: Models that support the integration of children with varied developmental levels. In C.A. Peck, S.L. Odom and D.D. Bricker (Eds.) *Integrating young children with disabilities into community programs: Ecological perspectives on research and implementation.* (pp. 83–107.) Baltimore, MD: Paul H. Brookes.

Roberts, J.E., Burchinal, M.R. & Bailey, D.B. (1994). Communication among preschoolers with and without disabilities in same-age and mixed-age classes. *American Journal on Mental Retardation, 99* (3), 231–249.

Rodd, J. (1996). *Understanding young children's behaviour.* Sydney: Allen and Unwin.

Rogers, C. (1951). *Client-centred therapy.* London: Constable.

Rogers, C.R. & Freiberg, H. (1994). *Freedom to learn.* (3rd ed.) Columbus, OH: Merrill.

Rogers, N. (1994). Foreword. In C.R. Rogers and H. Freiberg (Eds.) *Freedom to learn.* (3rd ed.) (pp. iii–vii.) New York: Merrill.

Rogers, W. (1994). *Behaviour recovery.* Melbourne: A.C.E.R.

—— (1998). *'You know the fair rule' and much more: Strategies for making the hard job of discipline and behaviour management in school easier.* Melbourne: A.C.E.R.

Rolfe, S., Lloyd-Smith, J. & Richards, L. (1991). Understanding the effects of infant care: The case of qualitative study of mothers' experiences. *Australian Journal of Early Childhood, 16* (2), 24–32.

Ronai, C.R. (1997). On loving and hating my mentally retarded mother. *Mental Retardation, 35* (6), 417–432.

Rose, S.R. (1983). Promoting social competence in children: A classroom approach to social and cognitive skill training. In C.W. LeCroy (Ed.) *Social skills training for children and youth.* (pp. 43–59.) New York: Haworth Press.

Rosenthal, D.M. & Sawyers, J.Y. (1996). Building successful home/school partnerships: Strategies for parent support and involvement. *Childhood Education, 72* (4), 194–200.

Rossman, B.B.R. & Rosenberg, M.S. (Eds.) (1998).The multiple victimization of children: Incidence and conceptual issues. In B.B.R. Rossman and M.S. Rosenberg (Eds.) *Multiple victimization of children: Conceptual, developmental, research, and treatment issues.* (pp. 1–5.) New York: Haworth Press.

Roth, R.A. (1989). Preparing the reflective practitioner: Transforming the apprentice through the dialectic. *Journal of Teacher Education, 40* (2), 31–35.

Rubin, Z. (1980). *Children's friendships.* Boston, MA: Harvard University Press.

Rutter, M. (1985). Resilience in the face of adversity: Protective factors and resistance to psychiatric disorder. *British Journal of Psychiatry, 147,* 598–611.

Ryan, N.M. (1989). Stress-coping strategies identified from school age children's perspective. *Research in Nursing and Health, 12,* 111–122.

Saifer, S., Clark, S., James, H. & Kearns, K. (1993). *Practical solutions to practically every problem.* Sydney: Pademelon.

Sainato, D.M. & Carta, J.J. (1992). Classroom influences on the development of social competence in young children with disabilities. In S.L. Odom, S.R. McConnell and M.A. McEvoy (Eds.) *Social competence of young children with disabilities: Issues and strategies for intervention.* (pp. 93–109.) Baltimore, MD: Paul H. Brookes.

Sameroff, A.J. (1990). Neo-environmental perspectives on developmental theory. In R.M. Hodapp, J.A. Burack and E. Zigler (Eds.) *Issues in the developmental approach to mental retardation.* (pp. 93–113.) Cambridge, UK: Cambridge University Press.

Sandall, S.R. (1993). Curricula for early intervention. In W. Brown, S.K. Thurman & L.F. Pearl (Eds.) *Family-centered early intervention with infants and toddlers: Innovative cross-disciplinary approaches.* (pp. 129–151.) Baltimore, MD: Paul H. Brookes.

Sandall, S.R. & Schwartz, I.S. (2002). *Building blocks for teaching preschoolers with special needs.* Baltimore, MD: Paul H. Brookes.

Sandler, A.G. & Mistretta, L.A. (1998). Positive adaptation in parents of adults with disabilities. *Education and Training in Mental Retardation and Developmental Disabilities, 33* (2), 123–130.

Sapon-Shevin, M. (1986). Teaching cooperation. In G. Cartledge and J. F. Milburn (Eds.) *Teaching social skills to children: Innovative approaches.* (2nd ed.) (pp. 270–302.) New York: Pergamon.

—— (1996). Beyond gifted education: Building a shared agenda for school reform. *Journal for the Education of the Gifted, 19* (2), 194–214.

—— (1999). *Because we can change the world: A practical guide to building cooperative, inclusive classroom communities.* Boston, MA: Allyn and Bacon.

Schaffer, H.R. (1998). *Making decisions about children: Psychological questions and answers.* (2nd ed.) Oxford, UK: Blackwell.

Schilling, R.F., Schinke, S.P., Blythe, B.J. & Barth, R.P. (1982). Child maltreatment and mentally retarded parents: Is there a relationship? *Mental Retardation, 20* (3), 201–209.

Sebastian, P. (1989). *Handle with care: A guide to early childhood administration.* (2nd ed.) Milton, QLD: Jacaranda Press.

Sekowski, A. (1995). Self-esteem and achievements of gifted students. *Gifted Education International, 10* (2), 65–70.

Seligman, M.E.P. (1975). *Helplessness: On depression, development and death.* San Francisco, CA: W.H. Freeman and Co.

Seligman, M. (1995). *The optimistic child.* Sydney: Random House.

Sharp, S. & Thompson, D. (1994). The role of whole-school policies in tackling bullying behaviour in schools. In P.K. Smith and S. Sharp (Eds.) *School bullying: Insights and perspectives.* (pp. 57–83.) London: Routledge.

Simons, J. (1986). *Administering early childhood services*. Sydney: Sydney College of Advanced Education.

Slaby, R.G., Roedell, W.C., Arezzo, D. & Hendrix, K. (1995). *Early violence prevention: Tools for teachers of young children*. Washington, DC: National Association for the Education of Young Children.

Smith, A.B. (1990). Early childhood on the margins. *Australian Journal of Early Childhood, 15* (4), 12–15.

Smith, M.A., Schloss, P.J. & Hunt, F.M. (1987). Differences in social and emotional development. In J.T. Neisworth and S.J. Bagnato (Eds.) *The young exceptional child: Early development and education*. (pp. 350–386.) New York: Macmillan.

Smyth, J. (1989). Developing and sustaining critical reflection in teacher education. *Journal of Teacher Education, 40* (2), 2–9.

Soden, Z. (2002a). Daily living skills. In L. Porter (Ed.) *Educating young children with additional needs*. (pp. 117–139). Sydney: Allen and Unwin.

—— (2002b). Daily living skills. In L. Porter (Ed.) *Educating young children with special needs*. (pp. 117–139). London: Paul Chapman/Thousand Oaks, CA: SAGE.

Sonkin, D.J. (1998). *Wounded boys; heroic men: A man's guide to recovering from child abuse*. Holbrook, MA: Adams Media Corporation.

Stainton, T. & Besser, H. (1998). The positive impact of children with an intellectual disability on the family. *Journal of Intellectual and Developmental Disability, 23* (1), 57–70.

Stanley, D. (1996). How to defuse an angry parent. *Child Care Information Exchange, 108,* 34–35.

Steele, B.F. (1986). Notes on the lasting effects of early child abuse throughout the life cycle. *Child Abuse and Neglect, 10,* 281–291.

Stoiber, K.C., Gettinger, M. & Goetz, D. (1998). Exploring factors influencing parents' and early childhood practitioners' beliefs about inclusion. *Early Childhood Research Quarterly, 13* (1), 107–124.

Stonehouse, A. (Ed.) (1988). *Trusting toddlers: Programming for one to three year olds in child care centres*. Watson, ACT: Australian Early Childhood Association.

—— (1991a). *Our code of ethics at work*. Watson, ACT: Australian Early Childhood Association.

—— (1991b). *Opening the doors: Child care in a multi-cultural society*. Watson, ACT: Australian Early Childhood Association.

—— (1994a). *Not just nice ladies: A book of readings on early childhood care and education*. Sydney: Pademelon.

—— (1994b). *How does it feel?: Child care from a parent's perspective*. Watson, ACT: Australian Early Childhood Association.

Swetnam, L., Peterson, C.R. & Clark, H.B. (1983). Social skills development in young children: Preventive and therapeutic approaches. In C.W. LeCroy (Ed.) *Social skills training for children and youth*. (pp. 5–27.) New York: Haworth Press.

Tannenbaum, A.J. (1983). *Gifted children: Psychological and educational perspectives*. New York: Macmillan.

Teyber, E. (1992). *Helping children cope with divorce*. San Francisco, CA: Jossey-Bass.

Thompson, B.J. (1993). *Words can hurt you: Beginning a program of anti-bias education.* Menlo Park, CA: Addison-Wesley.

Tizard, B., Philps, J. & Plewis, I. (1976). Staff behavior in pre-school centers. *Journal of Child Psychology and Psychiatry, 17* (1), 21–33.

Trawick-Smith, J. (1988). 'Let's say you're the baby, OK?': Play leadership and following behavior of young children. *Young Children, 43* (5), 51–59.

Trickett, P.K. (1998). Multiple maltreatment and the development of self and emotion regulation. In B.B.R. Rossman & M.S. Rosenberg (Eds.) *Multiple victimization of children: Conceptual, developmental, research and treatment issues.* (pp. 171–187.) New York: Haworth Press.

Turnbull, A.P. & Turnbull, H.R. III (1997). *Families, professionals and exceptionality: A special partnership.* (3rd ed.) Upper Saddle River, NJ: Merrill.

Tymchuk, A.J. (1992). Predicting adequacy of parenting by people with mental retardation. *Child Abuse and Neglect, 16,* 165–178.

van Boxtel, H.W. & Mönks, F.J. (1992). General, social, and academic self-concepts of gifted adolescents. *Journal of Youth and Adolescence, 21* (2), 169–186.

Veenman, S. (1995). Cognitive and noncognitive effects of multigrade and multi-age classes: a best-evidence synthesis. *Review of Educational Research, 65* (4), 319–381.

—— (1996). Effects of multigrade and multi-age classes reconsidered. *Review of Educational Research, 66* (3), 323–340.

Waters, J. (1996). *Making the connection: Parents and early childhood staff.* Melbourne: Lady Gowrie Child Centre (Melbourne) Inc.

Waters, M. & Crook, R. (1993). *Sociology one: Principles of sociological analysis for Australians.* (3rd ed.) Melbourne: Longman.

Webber, R. (1994). *Living in a step-family.* (2nd ed.) Melbourne: A.C.E.R.

Wells, R. (1997). *Helping children cope with divorce.* London: Sheldon.

—— (1998). *Helping children cope with grief: Facing a death in the family.* London: Sheldon.

Westberg, G.E. (1992). *Good grief.* (rev. ed.) Melbourne: Fortress.

Weyburne, D. (1999). *What to tell the kids about your divorce.* Oakland, CA: Harbinger.

Whelan, T. & Kelly, S. (1986). *A hard act to follow: Step-parenting in Australia today.* Melbourne: Penguin.

White, K.R., Taylor, M.J. & Moss, V.D. (1992). Does research support claims about the benefits of involving parents in early intervention programs? *Review of Educational Research, 62* (1), 91–125.

Wodrich, D.L. (1994). *Attention deficit hyperactivity disorder: What every parent wants to know.* Baltimore, MD: Paul H. Brookes.

Zentall, S.S. (1989). Self-control training with hyperactive and impulsive children. In J.N. Hughes and R.J. Hall (Eds.) *Cognitive-behavioral psychology in the schools.* (pp. 305–346.) New York: Guilford.

Zuckerman, B., Bauchner, H., Parker, S. & Cabral, H. (1990). Maternal depressive symptoms during pregnancy, and newborn irritability. *Journal of Developmental and Behavioral Pediatrics, 11* (4), 190–194.

Index